HEALTHY FOR YOUR LIFE

HEALTHY FOR YOUR LIFE

A holistic approach to optimal wellness

CARRIE DENNETT
MPH, RDN

othello press

othello press

OTHELLO PRESS
SEATTLE, WASHINGTON

Healthy For (Your) Life
www.healthyforyourlife.com

Published in the United States by OTHELLO PRESS
Trade Paperback ISBN 978-0-9997990-0-0

First Edition
Printed by CreateSpace, a DBA of On-Demand Publishing, LLC

Design by Jeff Paslay Designs: www.jeffpaslaydesigns.com
Cover illustration by Shutterstock

CONTENTS

Introduction   1

PART 1: WHO
Chapter 1   What is Health?   7
Chapter 2   Getting Launched   24

PART 2: WHAT
Chapter 3   Eating for Health   39
Chapter 4   Cooling the Fire of Inflammation   50
Chapter 5   The Power of Produce   67
Chapter 6   Staying Strong   77
Chapter 7   Fuel and Fiber   93
Chapter 8   The Flavor Factor   105
Chapter 9   Health Begins at Home   123

PART 3: WHEN
Chapter 10   Your Eating Day   135
Chapter 11   Finding the Time   144

PART 4: WHERE & HOW
Chapter 12   Intuitive and Mindful Eating   159
Chapter 13   The Journey Ahead   171
Chapter 14   Being A Savvy Nutrition Consumer   185

PART 5: WHY
Chapter 15   Head Games   197

             It's a Wrap   208
             Recipes   210
             Acknowledgements   217

Warming Up

DOES ANYONE READ BOOK INTRODUCTIONS? Thank you for reading this one, and I'll try to keep it brief, useful and to the point. This book was born out of the confusion I see every day in patients, friends, family and readers of my newspaper articles. Not just what to eat, but when to eat, how to eat and why to eat. And then there's the biggest mystery of all—who are we in relation to food? I totally understand that confusion, because, believe me, I've been there myself. We all swim in the same food and dieting culture, so it's hard to not be influenced by it to at least some degree.

When it comes to nutrition and food relationships, I'm a straight shooter (in other words, if a nutrition claim has no evidence to back it up, I'll say so), but I also know that nutrition, food and eating isn't black and white—not only do I see the many shades of gray, but I revel in them. When I'm working with patients one-on-one, I aim to help them find the nutrition path that's right for them, the one that leaves them feeling nourished and peaceful around food, with guidelines instead of rigid rules. I am SO anti rigid rules!

While reading this book isn't the same as meeting with me in person, I've tried to distill some of my best knowledge about nutrition and food relationships onto these pages. Because I'm just scratching the surface, I've included a robust resource list, and you'll find even more resources in an update-able list on the book website (www.healthyforyourlife.com), along with bonus worksheets and other materials.

Some of the worksheets include journaling exercises, and some readers may be wondering if they would benefit from keeping a food journal, especially if they are using this book to guide or inspire some changes to their food choices or eating habits. My answer is "maybe." I am a big advocate of keeping a "food and feelings" journal that tracks what and when you eat (without getting nit picky about amounts and definitely without tracking calories or grams of whatever), how your food makes you feel, and how you are feeling generally. Here are some elements that may be useful to log in a food and feelings journal:

- What you ate and drank (again, no tracking calories or macros)
- When you ate and drank
- How hungry you are when you started eating
- How full/satisfied you are when you finish eating
- Any cravings or non-hunger impulses to eat (boredom, stress, anxiety, etc)
- Bedtime and wake times
- How well you slept
- Type/amount of movement (aka physical activity)
- Any self-care habits you practiced
- General thoughts or observations about your relationship with food and your body

In my personal and professional experience, writing down this type of information is useful for two major reasons: it offers you an objective look at your eating patterns (our memories are not as reliable as we think), which can help you notice patterns that aren't serving you well (like going too long between meals, not eating enough protein, and so on) and it can help you be mindful as you start to form new habits. All of this requires honesty in your journal, of course, which in turn asks that you be compassionate towards yourself if you aren't thrilled with what your food journal reveals. Remember that awareness of our habits is a vital first step to moving forward and cultivating positive change. No one likes to be judged, so please don't judge yourself. You're trying to do your best—we all are.

It should be clear that this is not a diet book, but just in case—this is not a diet book. As I'll talk about, diets don't work, but that doesn't mean that you might not have food habits that aren't working for you. That said, if this book inspires you to make some changes—and I hope that it does—make those changes with sustainability in mind. In other words:

- Make changes at a pace that doesn't overwhelm you.
- Make changes that will enhance your physical and mental wellness.
- Make changes that you are confident you'll be happy to maintain for life (otherwise you will have turned this book into a diet).

In keeping with my journalistic nature, I've organized this book into five sections: who, what, when, where and how, and why. Those are the key elements of any news story, and the key elements of forming a healthy, nourishing relationship with food. And now, let's begin our story!

PART 1

Who

You are a unique individual,
and your path to health and well-being
will be equally individual.

CHAPTER 1

What is health?

IF YOU HAVE NEVER BEEN ON A DIET, you are a rare bird indeed. Odds are that you've been on at least one diet, even if it was to lose "just a few pounds" before a wedding, class reunion or beach vacation. Perhaps you are like many of the patients I see in my office, who have tried every diet out there, some of them more than once. The fact that they were sitting in my office served as testament to the fact that diets don't work.

No only do diets not work, but the extrinsic, artificial rules they impose get in the way of having a healthy relationship with food and physical activity. And when you have a healthy relationship with food and physical activity, your weight tends to settle at the place it is naturally meant to be. And that's a good thing, for both physical, mental and emotional health.

In this chapter, I'll talk about:

- Why it's time to move **beyond the dieting mentality**,
- Then I'll bust a few **weight loss myths** (I do love myth busting).
- After that, I'll talk a bit about **Health At Every Size**® (which contrary to what some critics say, does not mean that you are healthy no matter what size you are).
- Then I'll end the chapter by talking about **compassionate self-care.**

Moving beyond diets

YOU MIGHT NOT BE INTERESTED in losing weight, but if you are, one of the top questions on your mind is likely, "What's the best diet?" Low-carb (like Atkins or South Beach)? Paleo? Vegan? Low-fat (like Ornish or any holdover diet from the late 80s - early 90s)? The answer to that question is that it doesn't matter—research comparing various diets has shown time and time again that no particular diet is better for losing weight.

While there are some slight differences between studies, the big picture is this: for each diet studied, some individuals lose a significant amount of weight while others lose very little weight (even when they stick to the diet) but in the end the average results are the same (the end is usually 6 months after the end of the "actively dieting" part of the study).

This tells us two things:

1. You might lose more weight on a low-fat diet, but stall on a low-carb diet, while the opposite may be true for your spouse, best friend, coworker or cousin. As human beings, we are amazingly similar (your DNA is 99.9 percent the same as any other human being out there), yet as individuals we can be amazingly different in how our bodies and minds respond to food, activity and other contributors to health (sleep, stress, and so on).
2. The diets that produce the most average weight loss initially also have the quickest rebound effect (weight gain). By six months to a year after the study, the participants are all in the same weight boat (on average).

All that aside, there's a more significant bottom line: Diets don't work. By "don't work," I mean that even when people lose weight, they almost always gain the weight back, often with some extra pounds thrown in for good measure. In the short term, the diet may appear to be successful, because it did lead to weight loss. But who wants to lose weight only to gain it back? For weight loss diets to truly work, they would need to have a much better rate of long-term success (in other words, most dieters would need to keep off most of their lost weight for the rest of their lives). That simply does not happen, because our bodies have very powerful mechanisms for adapting to restriction of food and calories.

(Just to be clear, when I talk about "diet" in the context of "diets don't work" I'm talking about weight loss diets, specifically, not diet in the more general sense of "the sum of food consumed by a human or other organism.")

Most weight loss studies only follow up with participants for two years after the study is over. At that point, most lost pounds have returned due to a gradual weight regain that has no signs of stopping. Some studies have reported greater success with preventing regain when people participate in a high-intensity lifestyle intervention program for the long-term, but that's not something that's available to most people.

So what happens when you lose weight, regain it, lose weight again, regain it again, and so on, and so on? The evidence strongly suggests that you are likely to see your weight go up over time. The very act of dieting may, in the end, make weight gain more likely—especially if you diet when you are already a "normal" weight on the BMI charts.

Weight loss myths

DESPITE THE 95 PERCENT FAILURE RATE of weight loss diets, people continue to diet, and the weight loss industry makes tens of billions of dollars every year. One reason is that we keep buying into weight loss myths.

Myth 1: It's possible to lose weight and keep it off... you just have to find the right diet.
Fact 1: Diets do not work for long-term weight loss, regardless of what ratio of carbohydrates, protein and fat you eat or how many calories you consume. An estimated 95 percent of dieters regain their lost weight, and often gain additional weight. Many studies show that dieting itself is a strong predictor of future weight gain.

Myth 2: If you have enough willpower, you can lose weight and keep it off.
Fact 2: Willpower is a limited resource. It may help you some of the time, but it gets weaker the more you use it. For habit changes, effective strategies will get you much further than willpower, but even "strategic" attempts to lose weight will backfire when your body thinks you're starving.

Myth 3: If I want to lose weight, or keep it off, I need to pick a type of exercise that burns a lot of calories.
Fact 3: Using exercise as a weight loss "whip" is counter-productive on many levels. Regular physical activity is important for optimal health and wellness, but there are many ways to reap that benefit. When you choose forms

of physical activity that you enjoy and feels good to your body, you are more likely to engage in them regularly for the long term, and that brings the greatest benefits for both physical and mental health.

Myth 4: Diets may not work for long-term weight loss, but healthy lifestyle changes do.

Fact 4: "Healthy lifestyle changes" is often a secret code for "diet." If you are making healthy lifestyle changes for the sole purpose of losing weight, then you are dieting. It's a dirty little secret that the diet industry knows that "diet" has become a dirty word, and they are rebranding their programs as being about "health" or "wellness" or "lifestyle change." A wolf in sheep's clothing!

Myth 5: Losing weight improves health and prevents chronic disease.

Fact 5: It's true that obesity has been associated with many chronic diseases, including diabetes and heart disease, but association is not causation. In weight loss intervention studies that show improved markers of health (lower blood sugar levels, etc.) with weight loss, it's impossible to tell if it's the weight loss itself, or the increased physical activity and improved nutrition that are responsible for the change. Also, few studies factor in fitness levels, and no studies factor in the effects of weight stigma on health.

Many indicators of health, such as blood pressure, cholesterol levels and blood sugar or insulin resistance can be changed with healthy behaviors even if no weight is lost, and no study has ever shown that weight loss prolongs life.

We do know that body fat itself is metabolically active and can produce chemicals that encourage chronic inflammation throughout the body. Chronic inflammation contributes to heart disease, type 2 diabetes, cancer, arthritis and many other health conditions. However, we also know that a nutritious diet rich in vegetables, fruits and other plant foods, along with regular physical activity, helps reduce inflammation in its own right. On the other hand, we know that weight stigma increases stress, and stress contributes to inflammation, high blood pressure and other health problems.

Myth 6: My weight is determined by my genes.

Fact 6: Your genes determine the results of your food, exercise and other lifestyle habits. In studies where similar individuals eat food with identical calories and do identical exercise, they gain or lose differently. Ultimately, your body will do what it wants to do.

You can fight your body by restricting food and trying to pummel it into a certain shape with exercise, or you can love your body and nourish it with nutritious, delicious food, enjoyable movement and other types of compassionate self-care.

If you fight your body, you will be unhappy and your health will probably suffer. If you adopt self-care habits that make you feel good, even if you struggle a little bit with the change part at first (yes, change can be hard), your health and well-being will improve.

The Potential Perils of Yo-Yo Dieting

DIET, LOSE WEIGHT, REGAIN WEIGHT, repeat, repeat, repeat. Yo-yo dieting is an-all-too common phenomenon. More and more people are dieting—whether for weight loss or for "health"—even though most do not maintain their weight losses. This is unfortunate, because not only can yo-yo dieting lead to greater weight gain over time, but it may also put us in the path of heart disease and diabetes.

Even among people who lose a significant amount of weight—10 percent or more—roughly 8 in 10 will regain that weight within a year. But dieting and yo-yo dieting are not limited to people at higher weights. National Health and Nutrition Examination Survey (NHANES) data shows that the percentage of dieters who have weights in the normal range on the body mass index (BMI) chart is on the rise, currently almost 50 percent of women and 20 percent of men, while more than 10 percent of women with an underweight BMI report wanting to lose weight. Many adults, adolescents and children with normal or underweight BMIs diet because they feel pressure—internal or external—to be thinner.

Some of that external pressure may come from public health messages, with terms like "war on obesity" or "obesity epidemic." Many experts are concerned that an obsession with thinness slimness can backfire over the long-term, and that public health campaigns should ditch the focus on body weight and emphasize nutrition and physical activity for all.

Why yo-yoing happens

The very act of weight loss—especially the loss of muscle that accompanies all weight loss—triggers the body to fight back by increasing hunger, slowing metabolism and encouraging fat storage. This metabolic adaptation served our ancestors well during time of feast and famine, but not so much in today's modern food environment, which encourages weight gain in people who are genetically predisposed to it. Repeated dieting attempts do nothing to reduce this vulnerability. Restricting food increases its appeal, which can leads to overeating—or even binging—and then weight regain.

Instead, what happens is fat overshooting—regaining more fat than was originally lost. The body wants to regain lost muscle, but regains fat first, so the drive to eat and slowed metabolism continue until muscle regain is complete. Overshooting after each cycle of weight loss and regain can contribute to an overall increase in weight over time. In fact, a 2016 study in the journal Evolution, Medicine and Public Health proposed that the body's uncertainty about food supply—the body can't tell the difference between intentional dieting and unintentional famine due to food shortages—may cause it to store more fat each time food restrictions lift than it would if food intake remained steady.

The health effects of yo-yo dieting

Other research supports this idea. A 2015 article in the journal Obesity Reviews suggests that lean dieters are at greater risk for fat overshooting than those who are classified as overweight or obese. The lower a dieter's initial body fat percentage, the higher the proportion of muscle they lose and the higher the proportion of fat they gain. Over time, with continued yo-yo dieting, this may add up to a substantial increase in body fat. Two studies, in 2012 and 2013, of female twins found that the more frequent the cycles of yo-yo dieting, the greater the increase in body weight over time, especially among adolescents who start dieting at a lower BMI. What's notable about these twin studies is that they are able to compare what happens when two genetically identical people take different dieting paths.

What's more, yo-yo dieting in people who have BMIs at or below the normal range appears to increase risk of type 2 diabetes, high blood pressure and heart disease. What about people who start dieting at a higher body weight? Research is inconclusive, in part due to varying definitions of yo-yo dieting used in studies. Some dieters may have one large loss and regain, while others may experience several smaller loss-regain cycles.

Looking beyond dieting

One of the most meaningful changes we can make for health is a change in mindset—accepting that we don't have ultimate control over body weight. What we do have control over is choices. We also have the power to form new habit to replace habits that aren't serving us well. To start, identify what actions—or inactions—in your life are disappointing you and set your goals around new actions that are in alignment with the person you want to be. Not sleeping enough? Skipping workouts? You can change that. Frustrated with how much alcohol you drink or how much you eat out. You can change that, too. Just don't make habits solely about weight loss, because those types of habits rarely stick. Creat habits that bring joy and energy into your life, and help you every day.

5 reasons not to diet

BEFORE YOU SIGN ON for another a restrictive eating plan that's likely been designed by someone who doesn't even know you, here are five reasons why to opt out of diet culture.

1. **Diets don't work.** Anyone who says they have found the proven way to lose weight and keep it off is selling snake oil, and counting on repeat customers. When you restrict calories enough to drop below your body's natural setpoint weight range, your body will push back, triggering weight regain. Over time, repeatedly losing and regaining weight (yo-yo dieting) may leave you in a worse place healthwise than if you never dieted. This is a bitter pill, especially if better health is one of your motivations for losing weight.

2. **Weight does not equal health.** People can be healthy or unhealthy at both lower weights and higher weights. Even in research that shows an association between weight loss and improved health, it's unclear whether it's the weight loss that's actually responsible for better health, or the behaviors people adopt in an effort to lose weight, such as better nutrition and regular physical activity).

3. **Dieting gets in the way of lasting change.** In other words, it doesn't help you develop sustainable habits. When you treat nutrition and physical activity only as a means to weight loss, you're not likely to

eat well or be active if your attempts don't lead to the results you want—and you're more likely to return to old habits even if you do lose weight.

4. **Dieting takes up mental bandwidth.** Since most people feel there's not enough hours in the day, why spend precious time obsessively logging your food and tracking your calories or macros? Why exhaust energy worrying about whether the food at a restaurant or party fits your diet rules or beating yourself up because you ate a food that's not "allowed." You might think that weighing less will free you from body image concerns, but dieting to improve body image is futile, because any newfound self-esteem will evaporate when you regain the weight.

5. **Restriction can lead to binging.** Dieting and food restriction have been shown to increase the risk of binge eating. When you feel deprived, you're more likely to engage in compensatory overeating once you stop restricting. This restrict-binge cycle is the opposite of a moderate, balanced, peaceful approach to food and eating.

Ditching the diet? What to do instead

GIVING UP ONE HABIT without replacing it with something else can create an uncomfortable vacuum that may suck you back into the diet culture. Here are four things you can do to move towards health and away from dieting.

1. **Investigate intuitive eating.** Babies and very young children instinctively know when and how much to eat, based on innate hunger and fullness cues. We start to unlearn those cues once we're encouraged to eat "just three more bites" or to clean our plate—or are taught that there are "good" and "bad" foods. The good news is that intuitive eating is a skill we can learn again, and the outcome is far more fruitful than what comes from continuing to diet. The book "Intuitive Eating" by dietitians Evelyn Tribole and Elyse Resch provides the ultimate guide.

2. **Focus on wellness, not weight.** Embrace new hab-

its that are good for whole-body health regardless of whether they lead to a change in weight. Since it's pretty clear that exercise and nutrition by themselves improve health, why not just focus on building better habits on those fronts, letting weight take a back seat? Eating foods that provide balanced nutrition, taste good and leave you feeling good has inherent value. So does moving your body regularly in ways that feel good to you. So does getting enough sleep and managing stress. Research shows that a Health At Every Size (HAES) approach improves health regardless of weight.

3. **Cultivate body respect.** When you diet, you are trying to make changes from a place of body hatred. Why not work on making changes from a place of body respect and acceptance? Weighing less is not the path to happiness, and when you only feel good about your body when you're losing weight, that's a temporary body image boost. People who accept their size—regardless of what that size is—tend to take better care of themselves and enjoy better health.

4. **Say "no" to weight stigma.** Weight stigma, especially when you internalize it, is toxic for health. In fact, weight stigma alone may be responsible for most of the health problems that are typically ascribed to higher body weights. Why? Because people who take weight stigma to heart are less likely to seek preventive health care and more likely to engage in behaviors that harm health. We can all benefit from increasing compassion, acceptance and respect for all people, of all body sizes—including ourselves.

Looking beyond 'healthy weight' to simply health

IS IT POSSIBLE TO HAVE a body mass index (BMI) in the "obese" range and be healthy? It's true that so-called "obesity" has long been associated with cardiovascular disease, type 2 diabetes and several forms of cancer, but a lingering question is the degree to which "obesity" itself actually contributes to poor health. For every study suggesting that as BMI increases, the risk of chronic disease and early death also increases, there are others demonstrating that people can be healthy—or unhealthy—at any body weight.

For example, a study published in 2016 in *The Lancet* examined data from more than 10 million people from four continents and found that BMI outside the normal range—both underweight and overweight—was associated with an increased risk of poor health and early death. However, a similar study of more than 300,000 Korean adults, also published in 2016, concluded that metabolic health was more important than BMI when it comes to future health risk.

What is health?

Health can mean many things, but when researchers look at health vs. lack of health at higher body weight, they are generally looking at metabolic health, which is why you may see the term "metabolically healthy obesity." Metabolic health means not having cardiovascular disease or type 2 diabetes or their precursors, which include pre-diabetes, high blood pressure and high cholesterol.

While it's possible that genetics play a role in being healthy at higher weights, how we live matters, too. Health at higher weights is more common among younger women who eat a healthy diet, are physically active and have a higher socioeconomic status. Women are more likely to seek out preventive healthcare, and lower socioeconomic status affects the availability of resources that support a healthy lifestyle, including healthy food, walkable neighborhoods and access to healthcare.

What's clear is that health is not a given—it something that's ours to be lost or gained based on the sum of our daily actions. A healthful diet, regular physical activity and avoiding tobacco use are important for protecting health and preventing disease, regardless of body weight, but research shows that the majority of Americans are not hitting those marks.

Staying healthy for life

If you want to get healthy, be healthy and stay healthy, then focusing on health-promoting behaviors is far more important than worrying about BMI. One reason is that BMI isn't the best way of looking at weight. BMI can't tell the difference between body fat and lean muscle—or where body fat is distributed. Maintaining lean muscle is supports health, especially as we age. Excess body fat can increase the risk of chronic disease, but that largely depends on where that fat is located. Subcutaneous fat (fat under the skin) is thought to carry the least risk, while visceral fat (fat around the body's abdominal organs) carries more risk, and fat deposits in the liver and muscles carry the most risk.

As for whether weight loss improves health, that depends. For healthy individuals with BMIs in the "obese" range who have normal blood pressure, blood sugar and cholesterol levels, losing weight has not been shown to improve them further, and in some cases it actually contributes to unhealthy physical and psychological effects, including further weight gain.

One unfortunate finding of long-term research studies is that as many as half to two-thirds of healthy individuals with BMIs in the "obese" range eventually become unhealthy. While it's not clear why this happens, increasing age and decreasing physical activity are likely factors. You can't do anything about growing older, but you can make a point to stay physically active. Two other factors that don't receive nearly enough attention are weight stigma and socioeconomic status, which can be profound sources of stress. Stress contributes to the very health problems that increase risk of cardiovascular disease and diabetes.

The movement connection

Regular physical activity is vital for good health for people regardless of weight, but it also may also explain why higher body weight isn't always associated with metabolic health risks. Physical activity promotes stable blood sugar, blood pressure and cholesterol levels and helps maintain or build lean muscle, improving body composition. The research studies that actually consider fitness when looking at the connection between weight and health tend to find that healthy "obese" individuals are fitter than their unhealthy peers and have essentially the same risk of chronic disease and premature death as the healthy normal-weight participants.

Physical activity doesn't have to come from just gym workouts or other planned activity, either. Minimizing the amount of time spend sitting or otherwise being sedentary is a key difference between healthy and unhealthy "obesity." A 2015 study in the American Journal of Clinical Nutrition found that healthy "obese" individuals logged significantly more incidental activity—the type you get when you're walking to the office water cooler or puttering around the house instead of sitting on the couch—than unhealthy "obese" individuals, but that moderate-to-vigorous physical activity was about the same between groups.

Individuals are not statistics

Weight has become a handy-but-inaccurate shorthand for health. The truth is that having a BMI in the normal range doesn't automatically protect someone from developing health problems, and having a BMI in a higher range doesn't guarantee that someone is unhealthy or will become so. No matter what statistics say, what's important is your individual health status and the actions you take to improve or maintain that status.

Health at Every Size

HAVE YOU HEARD OF "HEALTH AT EVERY SIZE"? What ideas does it bring to mind? Some people think that Health At Every Size®, or HAES®, encourages a "heck with it all" mindset. That's not true at all. Many people also think that HAES® teaches that everyone is healthy at whatever body size/weight they are currently at. That's also not true.

What HAES® does say is that health and weight are two different things. You can have an "normal" BMI and be unhealthy, or you can be "overweight" and be healthy. Or vice versa. HAES® is about helping you be healthier at whatever size you are right now, while recognizing that health means different things to different people, and includes mental/emotional health as well as physical health.

If you want to be your healthiest, it's important to attend to not just nutrition and movement/exercise, but sleep and stress, too. When you focus on your mental and physical health and well-being, instead of on your weight, you start to bring your body and mind into balance. When we tend to our health through meaningful self-care instead of worrying about our weight, our bodies tend to find their natural, healthy weights because our bodies like to be in balance. What that weight will be is different for each person.

The principles of HAES

HEALTH AT EVERY SIZE® recognizes that weight does not dictate how healthy someone is, and that health is not all about personal responsibility. Embracing the principles of HAES® is good for every body of every size:

- **Weight inclusivity.** Accept and respect the inherent diversity of body shapes and sizes and reject the labeling specific weights as ideal/healthy or undesirable/unhealthy.
- **Health enhancement.** Support health policies that improve and equalize access to information and health services, as well as personal practices that improve human well-being. This includes paying attention to individual physical, economic, social, spiritual, emotional, and other needs.
- **Respectful care.** Acknowledge our biases, and work to end weight discrimination, weight stigma, and weight bias.

18

Provide information and services from an understanding that socio-economic status, race, gender, sexual orientation, age, and other identities impact weight stigma, and support environments that address these inequalities.

- **Eating for well-being.** Promote flexible, individualized eating based on hunger, satiety, nutritional needs, and pleasure, rather than any externally regulated eating plan focused on weight control.
- **Life-enhancing movement.** Support physical activities that allow people of all sizes, abilities, and interests to engage in enjoyable movement, to the degree that they choose.

Source: The Association for Size Diversity and Health (ASDAH)

"Body trust is not in any sense of the word a diet. Body trust is an internally directed process, a gentle way to care for yourself for the rest of your life. Trusting your body means getting in touch with inner signals and letting your body sort out the weight question itself."

— Dayle Hayes

Want to be healthier? Try a little tenderness

IF YOU THINK YOU NEED TO CHANNEL your inner drill sergeant in order to eat your vegetables and get to the gym, think again. Research shows that a healthy dose of self-compassion actually helps us form habits that support good health. In the past decade or so, numerous research studies have shown that self-compassion is important for mental and emotional health and well-being. Newer research is also finding that self-compassion is important for physical health.

What is self-compassion?

According to self-compassion researcher and Kristin Neff, author of "Self-Compassion: The Proven Power of Being Kind to Yourself," there are three elements to self-compassion. Mindfulness, which is being aware of negative thoughts, feelings and experiences without judging them or dwelling on them. Common humanity, or recognizing that we are all imperfect, and we all suffer. Self-kindness, which is showing yourself care and understanding when you experience those all-too-human imperfections.

The opposite of self-compassion is emotional reactivity, isolation, self-judgment and unhealthy perfectionism, all of which have been linked to depression, stress and reduced quality of life.

The stress connection

A 2017 study published in Health Psychology Open found that people who have higher levels of self-compassion tend to handle stress better—they have less of a physical stress response when they are stuck in traffic, have an argument with their spouse, or don't get that job offer—and they spend less time reactivating stressful events by dwelling on them. That's important, because not only does chronic stress directly harm health—the physical responses to stress include spikes in blood pressure and blood sugar along with suppression of the immune system—but if you react strongly to stress, you're more likely to employ unhealthy short-term coping mechanisms like smoking or numbing your feelings with food or alcohol.

The study also found that self-compassionate people are more likely to adopt health-promoting behaviors and maintain them even if they don't appear to be paying off in the short term. This may be especially important in the face of a health-related setback, like injury, illness or a disappointing lab result, because self-compassion takes the edge off negative emotions—fear, frustration, and disappointment—that might arise. This helps you continue to take good care of yourself instead of getting derailed.

Myths about self-compassion

Self-compassion often gets painted as selfish, lazy, or indulgent, but nothing could be further from the truth. People who are caregivers—by nature or circumstance—often find it difficult to offer themselves the compassion they freely give to others. However, connection with the rest of humanity is a core component of self-compassion, so to fully give to others, you need to give to yourself.

Are you a perfectionist? You may fear that if you are too nice to yourself you'll accomplish nothing. The truth is that when you make changes out of self-compassion, those changes are more sustainable than changes you make because you feel like you are unacceptable the way you are. You're also more likely to make daily choices that support long-term well-being, rather than indulging in short-term impulses. That may mean going for a walk instead of crashing on the couch, or putting down your fork when you're satisfied, not stuffed.

Research shows that self-compassion can increase motivation to change, possibly because it allows us to objectively evaluate areas for improvement and make changes without the threat of self-criticism. Lets say you have type 2 diabetes and your latest blood work shows that you haven't been managing your blood sugar well. Self-compassion will help you use that information to make changes to support better control going forward. Self-criticism can paralyze you, leaving you unable to change—and possibly ashamed to return to your doctor—leading to bigger health problems.

Becoming self-compassionate

Self-compassion should be easy, since we all want to be happy. Unfortunately—at least in some cases—we also want to avoid danger. In the face of true danger, we go into fight, flight or freeze mode. But when the "danger" is the uncomfortable emotions that rise from our inevitable mistakes or failures, our response can be self-criticism, self-isolation and self-absorption, which gets in the way of doing the things that will make us happier and healthier in the long run. Self-compassion helps us view uncomfortable emotions less of a threat.

So how do you cultivate self-compassion? Start with mindfulness. Unless you pay attention, you may be unaware of the thoughts that play and replay in your head. Practice observing your thoughts—are they compassionate, or critical? Be curious and non-judgmental—criticizing yourself for being self-critical adds insult to injury. Remind yourself often that to err is human, and to forgive, divine. Finally, show yourself kindness in ways that nurture mind, body and spirit. Take time to go for a walk, do some yoga, or prepare a nutritious meal. Incorporate activities that bring you joy, like reading a novel, puttering in the garden, or listening to favorite music. Strengthen connections with people important to you. Think love, not tough love.

Compassionate self-care

SELF-CARE IS ESSENTIAL to your health and well-being. Think of yourself as a plant, and self-care as the water that provides you with nourishment, helps you stay healthy and helps you grow and flourish.

These are the four categories of self-care:

Physical care
- Getting enough quality sleep
- Carving out time to rest and relax
- Eating energizing foods that also please your taste buds
- Moving your body in ways that feel good
- Appreciating your body, such as taking an aromatherapy bath or getting a massage

Emotional care
- Journaling about your thoughts and feelings
- Going on a date with your partner, or with friends
- Working with a therapist or life coach
- Saying kind things about yourself (positive self-talk)

Mental care
- Reading an interesting book
- Participating in a class or workshop
- Learning something new
- Engaging in a favorite hobby

Spiritual care
- Being in nature
- Meditating or praying
- Thinking about what you're grateful for
- Painting, dancing or drawing
- Volunteering

If you keep a journal, writing about the following questions can help you explore what self-care can bring into your life and motivate you to actually incorporate self-care into your life (a worksheet with these questions, and space for answers, is available on the website):

- What would your life look like if you were attuned and responsive to your needs?
- How would it feel to put yourself first and make your self-care a priority?
- How might your relationships change if you regularly took time for self-care?"
- "Which area of self-care—physical, mental, emotional or spiritual—do you most need to focus on right now?
- What specific steps can you take this month to make self-care a priority in that area?

At first making self-care a priority might be difficult. You might wonder if you really deserve it. Each of us deserves self-care right now, as we are today. You don't need to earn it by finishing a project, losing a few pounds, or waiting until your kids have moved out. Self-care isn't selfish. It isn't a luxury or an indulgence. Think of it as oxygen to your cells.

Chapter summary

I hope that you are thinking about the concept that health and weight are not one in the same (or, if you already have done some reading on this topic, I hope what you just read has bolstered that).

Here are the main takeaways from Chapter 1:

- Diets don't work.
- There are a lot of persistent myths about weight loss
- You can be healthy, or unhealthy, at any weight.
- Every body is worth of respect.
- You need compassionate self-care to thrive!

Coming up in Chapter 2, Getting Launched:

- Finding motivation for change
- Goals vs. outcomes
- Setting SMART goals
- Goals as affirmations
- Activity: Just three things
- The power of positivity

Getting Launched

ALL THE GOOD INTENTIONS in the world won't make a bit of difference if you aren't able to turn those intentions into actions. I saw a saying a few years ago that sums this thought up nicely: "If you reach too hard for the stars, you may never get off the ground." When you're at Point A, and want to get to Point B, sometimes you just need to start walking, one step at a time, rather than obsessing over which mode of transportation is "ideal."

In this chapter, I'll talk about:

- Finding **motivation for change,** and why it's OK to feel ambivalent about change.
- Then I'll fill you in on **setting SMART goals** so you actually have a roadmap for where you want to go.
- Next you'll reframe those **goals as affirmations,** so you can further get your brain in the game.
- Then you'll do the **"Just Three Things"** activity, so you always know what you can do, no matter what, to keep moving forward.
- Finally, I'll talk about the **power of positivity,** and how it can help "reprogram" your brain.

Finding motivation for change

WHEN WE THINK ABOUT MAKING CHANGES, most of us don't really consider all sides completely. Instead, we often do what we think we "should" do, avoid doing things we don't feel like doing, or just feel confused or overwhelmed and give up thinking about it at all.

Feeling ambivalent is a normal part of the process of making a change. Thinking through the pros and cons of changing and the pros and cons of NOT changing can help you decide whether to change at all. If you do decide to make the change, the fact that you fully considered both sides can help you "hang on" to your plan in times of stress or temptation.

Print out the Pros and Cons of Change worksheet from the website. Write down the change you want to make in the space provided, then complete the worksheet, listing the "good" and "not-so-good" things you can see about changing or not changing.

Goals vs. outcomes

MANY PEOPLE CONFUSE GOALS AND OUTCOMES, but they are quite different. You have direct control over progress toward your goals via the actions you take, but you don't have direct control over progress toward desired outcomes. Or, more specifically:

- Goals should be things toward which you can take direct, concrete action, like eating more fruits and vegetables or exercising daily.
- Outcomes are possible results of the actions you take toward your goals, such as increased energy or improved blood sugar. These are less predictable.

Setting goals is a key component of changing habits. Feel free to jump right in to goal setting with the goal-setting worksheets on the website, but if you don't feel 100 percent ready to go into goal-setting mode, that's OK. You may be experiencing some ambivalence, which is totally normal (as I just finished talking about).

What you can do instead is choose one tiny goal, one thing that you will do in the next 24 hours. It can be as simple as going for a short walk on your lunch break or stopping at the grocery store to buy some fresh fruit and veggies, because what's lingering in your produce drawer is looking sad and limp. Or, your goal could be to fill out the Pros and Cons of Change worksheet on the website, if you haven't already. It's a worksheet worth fill out, even if you already feel raring to go, but if something is holding you back from committing to positive change, you may especially benefit from it.

Setting SMART goals

Setting goals is an important part of making continual progress toward the vision you have for your health and well-being. But it's important to set your goals the right way...the SMART way. This will not only give you a better roadmap for the changes you want to make, but it will help you see clearly how much progress you are making.

- **Specific:** Write your goals as simply as possible while clearly defining what you are going to do. Make sure to include how, what and why.
- **Meaningful:** Your goals should be aligned with your values, or how you want to live and what you want to stand for.
- **Adaptive:** To the best of your ability, this course of action will make your life better.
- **Realistic:** Given the resources (time, money, health, skills) you have available to you right now.
- **Timeframe:** When do you want to achieve your goal? Short-term goals may be weekly or monthly, while long-term goals usually have timeframes of 6 months to a year.

Also think about what obstacles might get in your way (lack of time, other demands, difficult feelings or emotions) and how you might overcome them or work around them. This will help you craft better goals. For example, look at the difference between vague and specific goals:

- **Vague:** "I want to eat more regularly."
- **Specific:** "I want to stop skipping lunch."
- **Specific and measurable:** "I want to eat a nourishing lunch every day. I'll start by making a short list of places near work where I can go grab lunch, but after this becomes a habit I will start planning for lunches I can bring from home, and how I can do advance prep to make it easier."

Goals as affirmations

TURNING YOUR GOALS INTO AFFIRMATIONS can be a powerful tool to continue programming your brain for change. You can write any and all of your long-range and short-term goals as affirmations, but if you only choose one, your 12-week goal is the most important goal to focus on.

First, grab a piece of paper and write down why you want to reach your goal. What will reaching that goal do for you? What will be different when you reach it? How will your life improve when you reach it? Look at what you've written, and use that information to create your goal affirmation (below). For best results, your goal affirmation should be:

- Present tense (as if you've already achieved your goal)
- Personal (using the reasons that getting healthy and well is important to you)
- Positive (phrase it as what you want to gain, not what you want to avoid)

Examples:

"It's been 12 weeks since I started working toward my health and movement goals, and I'm feeling great. I feel stronger and I have so much more energy. I'm really looking forward to a fun, active summer with my family and friends."

"I've been eating more nutritiously and moving regularly for the last 12 weeks, and I just got lab results back from my doctor's office. My cholesterol and blood sugar levels are down, and my doctor is really impressed with what I've been able to do without medication, just by eating more nutritious meals and including some type of fun physical activity each day. Not only do I have more energy, but I'm setting a healthy example for my kids."

To make your goal affirmation more powerful, actively visualize yourself the way you want to be. When you visualize how it will feel to be healthier, stronger, and more energetic, you are reprogramming your self-image. This makes it easier to change your behaviors to be consistent with that new, healthier image.

Now it's your turn to turn your 12-week goal into an affirmation. Try writing it on a sticky note or an index card and keeping it where you will see it frequently.

Activity: Just three things

WRITE DOWN THREE "quick hit" actions you can take, starting today, or tomorrow at the latest, to improve your nutrition, fitness or other health-related factors. Just three things. They don't have to be big things. Here are a few examples to get you thinking:

1. Tune into hunger/fullness levels during meals.
2. Set an alarm on phone to remind me to eat lunch.
3. Meditate for five minutes each morning.

Only, don't write them that way. Write them like this:

1. I use my hunger and fullness cues to let me know how much food I need at each meal.
2. I get very busy at work some days, I'm grateful it's so easy to set an alarm on my phone (I like the harp sound) to remind me to stop and nourish myself mid-day.
3. Taking just five minutes each morning to meditate helps me feel centered and grounded before starting my day...many days I end up doing more than five minutes!

What you have here are affirmations. Now it's your turn. Grab some paper, or print out the worksheet from the website and write down three "quick hit" affirmations.

When you settle on your three "quick hit" affirmations and your bigger 12-week affirmation, and have them written the way you want them, copy them down on a 3x5 card, or a sticky note, or some piece of paper that's easy to carry in your wallet or post where you can see it easily. You're going to read these affirmations at least once a day. Ideally more!

Do you want to really, really go for it? Write out a copy of your affirmations every day. You don't have to keep the paper you copy them on...it's the physical and mental combination of the act of writing that will help burn your affirmations into your brain and make them part of you.

The power of positive programming

ROGER BANNISTER is the first person to officially run a mile in less than four minutes. Before he accomplished this feat on May 6, 1954, many "experts" believed that such a feat was impossible. However, not only did Roger Bannister accomplish the "impossible," but runners have shaved almost 17 seconds off his record in the decades since.

- So how did Roger Bannister do it? What changed on that day nearly 56 years ago?
- Did the laws of physics change? No.
- Did the human body change? No.
- What changed was that Roger Bannister believed that it was

possible to run a mile in less than four minutes, and made it his goal.

Once he had the belief and the goal, he figured out what he needed to do to reach his goal…and he did it. Do you believe you can reach your goal? What do you need to do to make it happen?

Reprogramming your brain's software

We know what a great piece of software (aka good programming) can do for our computer. Unfortunately, we probably also know what a virus (aka bad programming) can do for our computer. What kind of programming are you installing into your brain?

The more you practice something or tell yourself something, the deeper the "neural tracks" you lay down in your brain. The deeper the tracks, the easier it is to follow them in the future.

Think about something that you're good at. Odds are that you weren't quite so good at it the first time you tried it. But you kept at it, and it got easier, and you got better. The same is true for new-to-you health and self-care behaviors.

Examples of positive mental programming

"I can and will do what it takes to reach my goal of taking good care of myself!"

"I can reach and maintain my health and wellness goals if I make a realistic plan and commit to it. I know it won't always be easy, but the effort I put into my plan will be totally worth it when I reach my goals."

"OK, I ate my lunch completely mindlessly, but I can easily get back on track with my next meal. I can also come up with a few strategies for tuning in more to the experience of eating, even when I have no choice but to eat my meal quickly."

Examples of negative mental programming

"I want to in a way that really nourishes me, but I've never been able to stick to a plan. I doubt that whatever I try this time will work, either. If I do manage to eat better for a while, I'll probably fall back into my old habits, just like before."

"Crap, I'm done with my lunch already? I didn't notice anything past the first bite! Why can't I just pay attention when I'm eating? What is wrong with me? Stupid, stupid, stupid! I'll never be able to eat more mindfully, what's the point of even trying?"

Remember Roger Bannister? What if he had told himself that the "experts" were right—a man can't run a mile in less than four minutes? He certainly had ample opportunity for negative talk…he tried and failed to break that barrier many times before he succeeded. If he had chosen to adopt an "I can't do it" attitude, well, he would have been right. It would have been a self-fulfilling prophecy.

So, tell yourself you can do it (because you CAN!), make a plan, and stick with it. Each time you take an intended action (and say a little "hooray, me!"), the easier it will be to do it again, and again. And if you falter (as you will…you're human, after all), just start again. And again. And again.

> "The reason most people never reach their goals is that they don't define them, or ever seriously consider them as believable or achievable. Winners can tell you where they are going, what they plan to do along the way, and who will be sharing the adventure with them."
>
> — Denis Waitley

Invest in yourself, not a diet

WHEN IT COMES TO WEIGHT LOSS DIETS, there's nothing new under the sun. Any "lifestyle change" or "wellness" plan that comes with a list of rules and restrictions is a diet, regardless of what cloaking devices they deploy to persuade you that it's not. Investing in a new diet is like giving a loan that will never be repaid, because roughly 95 percent of dieters regain the lost pounds, with many ending up at a higher weight than where they started. On top of that, obsessing over the number on the scale will not only not lead to long-term behavior changes that help you feel good, it will probably actually make you unhappy. Why? Because the dieting mindset is rooted in body dissatisfaction and self-hatred.

How can you invest in yourself in ways that matter instead of jumping on another diet bandwagon? Approach changes you consider making from a place of self-love. Fully investing in behavior changes that are rooted in self-care, respect and acceptance will reap dividends for life. Think about it: when you love someone, you accept and care for them, flaws and all (and we all have flaws). For example, I love my 9-month-old golden retriever and care for him daily with food, exercise and lots of affection, even if I don't particularly like him when he's being naughty. What would happen if you treated yourself the same way?

Questions to ask yourself:

- What kinds of foods make me feel nourished, energetic and alert? Do I consistently have those kinds of foods in the house? If not, what's getting in the way (planning, shopping).
- Am I thoughtful about the food I eat or do I tend to eat on the fly, skip meals or eat mindlessly? How can I pay more attention so that I nourish myself better and enjoy my food more?
- What kind of movement (physical activity) do I enjoy? Are there types of activity I used to do happily, but stopped for some reason? Would I enjoy re-incorporating them? What type of movement have I always wanted to try, but never have? Salsa dancing? Bellydance? Yoga? Water aerobics? What's stopping me, and how can I overcome those obstacles?
- How much sleep do I need to feel my best? Am I consistently getting that much? If not, what can I do to change that? Do I need to develop a new pre-bedtime routine, or is it a more serious issue that I should discuss with my doctor?
- Do I like what I see when I look in the mirror? If not, is there anything I can realistically do to change what I see, or would I be better working on developing acceptance and respect?
- Am I in the habit of putting everyone (and everything) else first, before meeting my own needs? What would happen if you refilled your well regularly so you felt better physically and mentally?

Three more things:

- **Don't make everything about weight.** For example, exercise to be strong and flexible and have more endurance. Eat nutritious food because it helps you stay energized. Sleep because it feels good.
- **Declutter your media.** This includes magazines, email newsletters and social media feeds. Seeing constant reminders of health and body ideals that are unattainable for most

31

mortals can warp how you feel about nutrition and fitness—as well as how you see your own body and other people's bodies. These message can inspire "healthy hatred," or trying to make healthy changes from a place of self-hatred.

- **Get out of your comfort zone.** It can feel safe to stick with the tried-and-true, but we expand our world when we are willing to at least dip our toes beyond the edges of our comfort bubble. New foods, new ways to move, new ways to relax or be mindful. Curate the kind of life you want to live.

What would your future self say?

WE HUMANS TEND TO BE SHORTSIGHTED CREATURES, often acting to satisfy our immediate wants rather than our longer-term wishes. That may have served us well back in the days when we had to be on alert for saber-tooth tigers, but not so much today if you fancy the idea of living long and living well.

Do you tend to act without thinking, or do you use advance planning and forethought to guide your decisions? Some people are more wired to be impulsive than others, predisposed to quickly react to internal stimuli (like hunger or emotion) or external stimuli (like food advertisements, being in a food-related social setting, or simply seeing food) regardless of the consequences. When you frequently have impulsive reactions to food, this can work against what you really want for your health and well-being. Here are three tips to start making more thoughtful food decisions:

- **Practice mindful awareness.** In other words, if you are making an impulsive decision, be aware, in the moment, of what you are doing. Clearly and objectively seeing behavior patterns that aren't serving you is a necessary step in the path to change.
- **Avoid self-judgment.** It doesn't feel good to be judged. Self-judgment can lead you to stick your head in the sand and ignore the reality of the behaviors you would like to change. Everyone has something they would like to change—show yourself some compassion.
- **Shift your focus.** For example, weigh the immediate desire to finish the French fries with how you want to feel after the meal (intermediate desire) and what you want for your health (long-term desire).

I was explaining this concept to one of my tech patients once, and he said to me, "Oh, future self." Apparently, writing code for your "future self" is also a concept that web developers use, since writing convoluted code means their future self will have to struggle to read it. Considering what your future self would want you to do can also guide you to make in-the-moment choices that benefit long-term health:

- **Impulse:** Hit the snooze button instead of going for a walk. Think about how the walk will make you feel more energized and ready to tackle your day, and how regular, consistent physical activity will help you stay strong and vital with age.
- **Impulse:** Dine out instead of cooking a healthy dinner. The more you eat out, the harder it is to eat healthfully, so consider the long-term effects of acting on this particular impulse frequently. Also, consider the financial impact.
- **Impulse:** Grab a doughnut from the office break room (which you only spotted because you were refilling your water glass). Think of the benefit of avoiding a sugar crash, maybe choosing a more nutritious snack if you are actually hungry. Remember that there will be sweet treats in your future, if you choose. Why not save that indulgence for a time when you can plan for it and really sit and enjoy it?

Another patient once told me how well this works for her, much to her surprise. When she feels the impulse to keep eating delicious food even though she's getting full, or skip cooking in favor of takeout, she thinks about how she wants to physically feel afterwards. This guides her to make decisions that ultimately serve her health and well-being, without feeling deprived. Making choices for the long-term does not have to mean being miserable in the moment!

Chapter summary

I hope that you are thinking about the concept that health and weight are not one in the same (or, if you already have done some reading on this topic, I hope what you just read has bolstered that).

Here are the main takeaways from Chapter 2:

- It's okay to feel ambivalent about changing.
- Setting goals is key to reaching your desired health and well-being outcomes.
- Turning goals into affirmations makes them more "real."

Coming up in Chapter 3, Eating for Health:

- Is there a "healthiest" diet?
- Plant-based eating
- Energy density
- Can you disease-proof yourself?

PART 2

What

You are so much more than what you eat, but what you eat can help you be your best self and live your best life.

Eating for Health

DO YOU FEEL LIKE you have nutrition whiplash trying to figure out how you should feed yourself if you want to be healthy and stay well? I don't blame you! By the end of this chapter, you'll feel clearer about what it means to eat nutritously, and why there's no such thing as one perfect or "magic" diet. It will open the door to a more relaxed way of eating, as well as inspiration for making your own eating better every day.

In this chapter, I'll talk about:

- Why the **healthiest, most nutritious way to eat** may be different for you than for anyone else.
- However, the most nutritious ways of eating do have some things in common, so I'll fill you in on the benefits of **plant-based diets**, and why they don't mean you have to only eat plants (unless you want to).
- Then I'll talk about he difference between **energy density and nutrient density**, and why you want more of the second, less of the first.
- Finally, I'll go into myth-busting mode to let you know why you can't **"disease-proof"** yourself.

What's the healthiest way to eat?

WHAT'S THE HEALTHIEST WAY TO EAT? That depends on who you ask. At times, it may seem like everyone from your neighbor to your coworker to the latest best-selling diet book author claims to know the One Perfect Way to eat for weight loss or health, but odds are that these dietary advocates disagree with each other in some fundamental ways. So, who's right…and who's wrong?

The truth is this: There is no one single way to eat for nutrition and better health, no one perfect diet. When someone sings the praises of a specific way of eating, they may have found the pattern that works best for them, and it probably works really well for some other people, too. But that doesn't mean it will work for everyone.

As a species, we humans are quite similar on a cellular and genetic level, yet as individual specimens we can be amazingly diverse. That's why your neighbor may have endless energy on a vegan diet while a Paleo diet makes your coworker feel like they're on top of the world. Ironically, these two dietary patterns appear to be polar opposites: The Paleo diet includes meat but excludes grains and legumes, while the vegan diet includes grains and legumes but excludes meat and other animal products. How can both diets work? The answer lies in what they have in common.

What nutritious diets have in common

What does a nutritious way of eating look like? The most nutritious, health-promoting eating styles generally minimize processed foods while containing a variety of whole plant foods. In other words, a plant-based diet.

I know Paleo dietitians and vegan dietitians who eat wonderfully nutritious, balanced diets. Their food provides high-quality fuel for their bodies, but they also enjoy what they eat. Yes, their diets have some big differences, but they have two huge similarities: They include lots of plant foods (especially vegetables) and they minimize highly processed foods.

Lots of plant foods and fewer highly processed foods. Those are the common denominators of a nutritious diet. From there, you can fill in the blanks to suit your taste buds and unique physiological needs by adding your choice of quality fats (nuts, seeds, avocados, olive oil, fatty fish) carbohydrates (whole grains, fruit, starchy root vegetables) and plant- or animal-based protein (legumes, soy, fish, sustainably raised meat, poultry, eggs, dairy).

We need a varied diet in order to get the vitamins, minerals, fiber and phytonutrients required for optimal health and wellness—optimal meaning what's possible for you based on your specific age, genetics, and health history, as well as your ability and interest in attending to your health— but there are endless combinations of foods that will get us to that goal. While we all need carbohydrates, fat and protein, there is no "magic" ratio that we should be striving for.

The nutritional big picture

When working with clients, I see problems arise when they focus on what they DON'T eat (like meat or grains), instead of being thoughtful about what they DO eat. Failing to see the big nutritional picture can easily lead to a "healthy diet" that isn't so healthful, after all. For example, a Paleo diet that includes lots of processed meats, Paleo cookies and coconut milk ice cream with very few vegetables isn't terribly nutritious. Neither is a vegan diet that is low on veggies, high on white bread, pasta, vegan cookies and soy ice cream.

Taken to extremes, fixating on avoiding meat or sugar or gluten can make us dogmatic about how we eat, even turning our food choices into a core element of our identities. ("You are what you eat" shouldn't be taken literally.)

An intuitive approach

It's a wonderful thing that there are many ways to eat healthfully and well, but it means that to find your optimal way of eating, you need to trust your body to tell you what that diet looks like. For many of us, it can be hard to relearn this intuitive approach, which we all had when we were small children! (We'll cover this in depth in Chapter 12.)

To start, let yourself choose from a wide variety of foods, and pay attention to how you feel. Do you feel energized for hours when you eat oatmeal for breakfast, or do you need more protein from, say, eggs or Greek yogurt? Do you run best on three square meals a day, three meals plus snacks, or six mini meals? Do you feel energized after eating meat, or tired? Are there certain "healthy" foods that make you feel bloated? Then they probably aren't healthy foods for you!

Keep in mind that while it may feel easier to simply adopt a ready-made dietary formula, it's rarely sustainable or satisfying. Investing in yourself by learning how to forge your own personal, intuitive path can help you enjoy the act of eating while realizing improved health and wellness for the rest of your life. It's about finding that sweet spot between eating to live and living to eat.

"To be nobody but yourself — in a world which is doing its best, night and day, to make you everybody else — means to fight the hardest battle which any human being can fight; and never stop fighting."

— E.E. Cummings

The benefits of loving your food

HOW DO YOU VIEW FOOD? Is it fuel, is it pleasure, or is it a bit of both? I've had spirited debates with people who firmly believe that food is supposed to be fuel—period—and that to view food as pleasure at all was a gateway to food addiction.

We are genetically hardwired to seek pleasure, because that's what helped our species survive back in the day. In today's health- and weight-centric culture, however, pleasure gets a bad rap—ironic, given that the modern food environment heavily promotes indulgent and less-nutritious foods. When we feel conflicted or confused about our food choices, rush through our meals, eat while distracted, we deprive ourselves of food pleasure and eating satisfaction. This can have negative consequences for health. But you can—and should—eat for both nutrition and pleasure.

Pleasure and nutrition: perfect partners

Obviously, food is fuel for your body, and filling your tank with the quantity and quality of food your body needs will help you operate at your best—"running on fumes" or regularly filling up with foods that are low on nutrition will leave you feeling lackluster. But food is also pleasure. If nothing else, this is true from a pure neurobiology standpoint—our brains are wired to register pleasure when we have experiences that we need to repeat in order to survive. If food didn't provide pleasure, we wouldn't exist today, because our caveman ancestors would have little motivation to put in the required effort needed to hunt a woolly mammoth and sleuth out roots and berries that weren't poisonous.

Unfortunately, our brain's reward circuitry doesn't always mesh well with the abundance of highly palatable food in today's modern food environment—especially if you find yourself stretched so thin with work-home-life responsibilities that the only pleasure you feel you have time for is food. After all, we all need to eat, and as one of my patients pointed out to me, you can eat chocolate while doing the laundry.

The key is to find balance. Taking food as fuel and deriving no pleasure from the experience is joyless, but if food is your primary source of pleasure, it's easy to veer into overindulgence. Using food as a primary source of pleasure can be like a canary in a coalmine—as sign that deeper needs aren't being met. However, when food is just one of many things that brings you pleasure, this can lead to better-for-you choices, because ultimately we want our food to taste good and leave us feeling good. It's not terribly pleasurable to end a meal feeling like you're full-to-bursting and halfway to a food coma—the antithesis of pleasure.

What makes a food pleasurable? Taste is obviously one factor, but it's also about what would feel good in terms of temperature, texture and substance. The crispiest, juiciest, most flavorful apple in the world won't bring you true pleasure if you're hungry for a warm, filling meal. Similarly, if you are craving a big salad but all that's available to you is a burger, you're not going to take a lot of pleasure in your meal.

Most people find a variety of foods pleasurable, and some of those foods are going to be more nutritious than others. Marrying pleasure and nutrition often takes some thought, both about what you would like to eat and where and how you are going to procure it. This is true whether you are cooking at home or sleuthing out suitable restaurant options. A good place to start is to experiment with some tasty new vegetable recipes at home or check out farm-to-table type restaurants that are doing interesting things with seasonal vegetables.

Is food your religion?

IN HIS 1825 BOOK, "The Physiology of Taste," Jean Anthelme Brillat-Savarin famously wrote, "Tell me what you eat, and I will tell you who you are." In modern times, that saying has morphed into "You are what you eat." Food is more than just fuel for our bodies—it has meaning and ritual, it evokes memories and emotions. Think of Sunday dinner (or Sunday brunch), think of holiday meals. In this way, food rightly becomes part of our identities, part of what makes us who we are. But what if we identify too strongly with how we eat?

Just as there are differing religious ideologies, there are differing dietary ideologies, and in our increasingly secular society, our dietary beliefs can become as dogmatic as those of any religion. In his 2015 book "The Gluten Lie: And Other Myths About What You Eat," religious scholar Alan Levinovitz, PhD, discusses how many of our food and nutrition beliefs are based on superstitions and magical thinking, leading to a faith-based view that's more religion than science.

Levinovitz points out that demonization of specific foods or food groups is cyclical, with some foods falling out of favor repeatedly over the centuries. Carbs, fat, meat, alcohol, MSG, gluten. This often leads to the belief that if excessive amounts of a certain food isn't good for you that even a small amount is health-wrecking. Take sugar: yes, it's a source of empty calories that, in excess, could contribute to health problems, but the calling it "metabolic poison" or comparing it to cocaine? That's a little over-the-top.

Pick pretty much any religion or fad diet and you'll find certain elements in common. Strict guidelines. Good and bad behaviors. The promise of personal transformation. The threat of temptation. Resist temptation and feel virtuous or even "pure." Succumb to temptation and feel guilty because you've sinned. To seek absolution, you may confess your sins to fellow believers.

A rigid eating plan is difficult to adhere to day after day. This can produce rigid one-track-mind thinking, because if you are working that hard you want to believe it's for a good reason. It can also lead to proselytizing—if you can convert others to your dietary bandwagon, this reinforces your beliefs and gives you a sense of belonging. Unfortunately, this can also alienate people. I have patients who tell me they avoid sharing meals with dieting friends or family members because hearing recitations of how many carbs or calories are in every food gets annoying, fast.

As an antidote to Brillat-Savarin, I offer these sage words from the philosopher Epictetus, who was born in AD 55: "Preach not to others what they should eat, but eat as becomes you, and be silent." Eat as becomes you. A novel idea, but a good one. The truth is that even ways of eating that have been shown through both time and scientific research to promote good health—such as the Mediterranean diet—have variability. The Mediterranean is a big area, after all, with many diverse food cultures.

If there's no one right way to eat, why are so many people so rigid in their diet beliefs? Possibly because, as a newish country, we don't have a strong traditional food culture, unless you count eating on the run. We also tend to be impulsive in our food choices, deciding what to have for dinner when standing in the grocery store at 6 p.m. Perhaps we adopt rigidity to avoid chaos, even though both are dysfunctional in their own way. When we adopt rigid diet rules, we set ourselves up for failure when a forbidden food crosses our lips due to circumstance or our inner rebel. This restriction can end up leading to chaos, with the idea that, "If I've sinned a little I might as well sin a lot."

To eat as becomes you, to find a middle ground between rigidity and chaos, you have to learn to trust your instincts and inner wisdom more than you trust the latest headline or best-selling book. Draw from on your own traditions, likes and dislikes. Expand your kitchen skills. Practice mindfulness. Eat your vegetables—and some dessert.

Plant-based diets

SO, IF YOU DECIDE TO EAT A PLANT-BASED DIET, does this mean you need to become a vegan or vegetarian? No, it doesn't! A plant-based diet means that you are filling most or even all of your plate with plant foods (fruits, vegetables, whole grains, nuts and seeds, herbs and spices), but there is more than one way to do this.

- **Vegan** includes no animal foods (even honey, which comes from bees).
- **Vegetarian** includes dairy foods and/or eggs but no meat, poultry, fish or seafood.
- **Lacto-ovo vegetarian** includes both dairy (lacto) and eggs (ovo).
- **Lacto-vegetarian** includes dairy but no eggs.
- **Ovo-vegetarian** includes eggs but no dairy.
- **Pescatarian** includes dairy foods and/or eggs plus fish and seafood (mostly for the healthy omega-3 fatty acids and an additional protein source), but no meat or poultry.
- **Flexitarian** includes dairy foods and/or eggs as well as small amounts of meat, poultry, fish and seafood. This is also known as a semi-vegetarian diet.
- **Healthy Omnivore** includes animal foods more liberally in the diet, but includes lots of plant foods and may frequently include vegetarian meals (Meatless Monday, for example).

If you take stock of your current way of eating and notice that you eat a lot of animal foods, and you would like to shift in the direction of a plant-based diet, a good place to start is to think of meatless meals you are already familiar with. Some examples might be bean or lentil soups or chilis, vegetarian lasagna, bean & veggie burritos, veggie stir-fries, veggie burgers, and so on. Grab a pen and paper and jot down a few ideas.

Some people worry that a vegetarian diet will be lacking in certain key nutrients, but the fact is that plenty of people who eat meat are lacking in certain key nutrients, especially if they rely heavily on fast food and other heavily processed foods! Whether or not you choose to eat meat and other animal foods, eating a variety of whole and minimally processed foods, with an emphasis on plant foods, will provide you with a good mix of the vitamins, minerals, phytonutrients and fiber that are essential for optimal health and well-being. Remember, it's about what you are eating, not just what you aren't.

What does science say about the benefits of a plant-based diet?

Naturally, if you make a point to shift your current eating pattern to incorporate more plant foods, you'd like to know how it will benefit you. Fortunately, there's been a lot of research looking at the health of populations who eat plant-based diets, as well as detailed laboratory research looking at the effects of certain compounds in plant foods (phytonutrients) on our bodies. From that, we know that plant-based diets:

- Promote general health
- Reduce the risk of some cancers
- Reduce the risk of cardiovascular disease and diabetes
- Tend to be higher in nutrients, lower in calories (i.e., nutrient-dense)

As an added benefit, eating a diet with more plant foods and fewer animal foods reduces your carbon footprint, if that's important to you.

Benefits of herbs and spices

Another concern can be that plant-based diets are bland. Not so! It's true that there is a certain savory aspect to meat and poultry that is harder to replicate with plant foods (although sautéed or roasted mushrooms can add a wonderful "meaty" quality to pasta sauces, veggie stirfries, and other dishes…they even make a good side dish on their own) but we can take a lesson from the many world cuisines that are plant heavy AND make ample use of herbs and spices.

We'll talk more about this in Chapter 8, but herbs and spices are more than just a great tool to make your meals delicious, they are also nutrient powerhouses in their own right (just chock-full of phytonutrients and antioxidants! They make meals more pleasurable, and can reduce the need to add sugar or salt to your dishes. Are you thinking, "But I don't like spicy food"? Never fear…most spices are not spicy HOT. If it's the spicy heat you don't care for, simply stay away from chile peppers and chile powder (including cayenne and chipotle). Problem solved.

Energy density

IS YOUR DIET ENERGY DENSE, OR NUTRIENT RICH? As a society, the answer is definitely energy-dense (energy is another term for calories, because calories are what we convert to energy). Overall, we eat few nutrient-rich vegetables and fruits but a lot of energy-dense refined grains, fats and sweets—in other words, foods that have more calories per bite, which you may or may not need.

Nutrient-rich foods are high in the nutrients we need more of for good health, like fiber, vitamins and minerals, and low in those we need less of, like salt, sugar and unhealthy fats. Non-starchy vegetables are the most nutrient-rich, followed closely by fruit. Next are legumes (beans and lentils), nuts and seeds, then eggs. After that, you have meat and poultry, milk and dairy, and grains. Not all foods within a group are equal: For example, whole grains, plain yogurt and lean meats are more nutrient-rich than refined grains, sweetened yogurt and fatty cuts of meat.

Can a food be both energy-dense and nutrient-rich? Sometimes. If you want to reduce the energy density of your meals, lowering fat isn't necessarily the best road to health, because many fats (nuts and seeds, avocados, olives and olive oil) have health benefits. You just don't want to make an entire meal out of them!

Instead, add more vegetables and fruits. Vegetables and fruits are tops for nutrient-richness because they are full of fiber and water, along with all those fabulous vitamins, minerals, antioxidants and phytonutrients. Here are a few ways to bump up the nutrients in your favorite meals:

- When doing the traditional protein + starch + veggie, fill half your plate with veggies. Including a cooked non-starchy veggie and a green salad is an easy way to do this.
- Add more veggies to soups, stews and meat-based pasta sauces.
- Add chopped or shredded vegetables to scrambled eggs.
- Add finely chopped mushrooms (which have a "meaty" flavor of their own) to burgers and meatloaf.
- Eat more broth-based soups and moist casseroles with lots of vegetables.
- Swap veggies for some of your starches and grains. Buy a spiralizer, and embrace the zoodle (zucchini noodle) where it make sense (I personally have some pasta sauces that it would be criminal to not put on actual pasta, and some where, I'm like, "Nah, I just need something to put the sauce on so I'm not just eating sauce.")
- Make stir-fries with tons of veggies and a healthy portion of protein (beef, chicken, fish, tofu or tempeh). You might not need the rice.
- Toss your favorite sandwich fixings on top of salad greens, instead of between two slices of bread.
- Use fruit for snacks. Have an apple and a small handful of nuts rather than just a large handful of nuts.

Can you disease-proof yourself?

AS MUCH AS WE HEAR that American is a junk food nation, many people do make eating healthfully a priority. When you believe in the power of good nutrition, it's easy to also believe that you can disease-proof yourself if you are sufficiently dedicated to eating your broccoli. Now, there are many good reasons to eat broccoli. It's delicious, especially roasted, and it's full of vitamins, minerals, antioxidants and phytonutrients. However, eating broccoli every day isn't going to turn you into a disease-free centenarian, even if you pair it with wild salmon and a salad made of goji and acai berries.

The idea that we can use diet and lifestyle to dodge all illness is appealing. The reality is that while eating well and maintaining other health-promoting habits reduces your risk of disease and untimely death, it can't wipe away all risk. Genetics and social factors—income, living environment, relationships, stigma and oppression—also affect health. The good news is that what you need to improve your health odds is less than what you might think.

The four crucial habits are eating at least five servings of fruits and vegetables per day, exercising at least three times per week, drinking alcohol in moderation and not smoking. People who have all four habits have the lowest risk of dying before their time, and that risk is the same regardless of body weight. Similar research in the United Kingdom has found that having all four healthy habits may equal an extra 14 years of life.

Barring addiction or severe physical limitations, those four habits are achievable for most people without massive effort. No radical restrictive diets or obsessive fitness regimes needed. What then, to make of health-improvement "projects" that do include rigid diets and excessive exercise? It's a side effect of healthism.

Healthism is the idea that we have a duty to be healthy, and that you can judge someone's health based solely on their behavior or appearance. The kind of nutrition and physical activity that promotes good health and longevity is not necessarily the kind that will promote the type of extremely fit appearance seen on cover models of health and fitness magazines.

Beware the mental trap of, "The more I exercise and the more perfectly I eat, the healthier I'll be and the longer I'll live." Too much of a good thing isn't necessarily better. Chasing impossible health ideals that are largely appearance-based can suck up time and mental energy that would benefit you more if used elsewhere. Even worse, there's a dark side. Some of those super-fit models on magazine covers have eating disorders, and eating disorders can be fatal. Don't judge a book by its cover.

What to do instead? Go for a walk. Or take a salsa dance class. Or do some yoga. Or find an indoor pool and go for a swim. Or visit a farmers market?

Chapter summary

I hope this chapter helped dispel a bit of the conflicting dietary dogma that often leads to nutritional whiplash! The core elements of a nutritious, health-promoting way of eating really aren't so complicated or change-able, contrary to what the diet book du jour or the latest headlines might say.

Here are the main takeaways from Chapter 3:

- There's no one way to eat healthfully.
- Invest in your health, not diets, but don't be dogmatic!
- You can't go wrong by eating lots of plants.
- It's great when your food is rich … nutrient rich!
- Yep, we really can't disease-proof ourselves

Coming up in Chapter 4, Cooling the Fire of Inflammation:

- What is inflammation?
- Glycemic index
- Your gut microbiota
- The Mediterranean diet
- Anti-inflammatory diets
- Anti-inflammatory powerhouses
- Food sensitivities

Cooling the Fire of Inflammation

ODDS ARE YOU'VE HEARD ABOUT INFLAMMATION, but you might not be sure of what it exactly is, or what it might mean for your health. I'll tell you what you need to know, straight up, without any gimmicks (this is important, because inflammation is a hot topic right now, and a lot of information out there is, to put it diplomatically, not quite accurate).

In this chapter, I'll talk about:
- **What inflammation is,** and why it's not always a bad thing (the key is whether it's acute inflammation or chronic inflammation).
- Then I'll give you a user-friendly explanation of the **glycemic index,** and why even though it can guide you to make more healthful food choices, you shouldn't treat it as gospel.
- It's impossible to talk about inflammation without talking about your **gut microbiota.**
- Then I'll talk about the **Mediterranean diet,** and why it's a good model for how to eat.
- Next I'll go a little deeper into the components of an **anti-inflammatory diet.**
- While healthful diets are about the sum of many parts (rather than a handful of "magic" foods), there are some foods that can rightly be called **anti-inflammatory powerhouses.**
- Do you wonder how **food allergies, intolerances or sensitivities affect inflammation?** I'll end the chapter with a quick overview.

What is inflammation?

INFLAMMATION SOUNDS BAD, BUT IS IT? Yes and no. Inflammation is one of your body's powerful healing processes. Under normal conditions, it's an acute (short-lived), controlled response to an injury, such as a cut or a sprain, or routine viral illnesses like colds and flu. Acute inflammation is responsible for healing damaged tissue and cleaning out waste products caused by the damage. It's a healthy, orderly process that defends your body until the crisis is over and you're on the mend.

Chronic inflammation, on the other hand, is an unhealthy, chaotic process that keeps going because the body's crisis doesn't end. It's the result of subtler insults to your body, including:

- Unhealthy diet
- Sedentary lifestyle
- Excess body fat
- Regular exposure to cigarette smoke or environmental toxins
- Excessive or unmanaged stress
- Lack of sleep
- Certain lingering health conditions (including inflammatory bowel disease)
- Age

Research suggests that chronic inflammation may be the root of many complex diseases, including heart disease, type 2 diabetes and cancer. Growing scientific evidence also suggests that diet and lifestyle can either create a pro-inflammatory environment (increasing inflammation) or an anti-inflammatory one (reducing inflammation).

What type of diet promotes (increases) inflammation?

The type of diet that encourages health-damaging chronic inflammation is, perhaps not surprisingly, the type of diet that most people would agree is less-than-healthful in general. Specifically, a diet that promotes chronic inflammation is:

- High in refined carbohydrates (white flour and products made from it)
- Low in fiber (from eating a lot of refined carbohydrates and few vegetables, fruits, whole grains and beans)
- High in saturated and trans-fats (trans-fats are also known as partially-hydrogenated oils)

51

A diet that encourages inflammation also contains:

- Excess sugar (this includes desserts, calorie-containing beverages as well as sugar that is added to many processed foods)
- Excess animal protein
- Excess alcohol
- Excess caffeine
- Low levels of vitamins, minerals and antioxidants
- Excess calories

Why excess calories? Simply put, eating to the point of overfullness is associated with an increase in inflammation. While one extremely large meal results in a temporary increase in inflammation, when this happens regularly, the inflammation can become chronic.

Glycemic index

CURRENT RESEARCH SUGGESTS — and many health experts argue — that choosing lower-glycemic foods may help prevent some chronic diseases, and the inflammation connection is likely to be part of the reason. That means an anti-inflammatory diet is based on foods that have a lower glycemic index.

The glycemic index ranks foods on a scale of 0 to 100 based on how much they raise blood sugar (glucose) levels in the few hours after a meal. Foods with a high glycemic index (above 70) are digested faster, so they cause sharper spikes in blood sugar. While the glycemic index can offer clues to what carbohydrate foods are healthier, the glycemic load is more applicable:

- **The glycemic index (GI)** tells you how quickly a set amount (50 or 100 grams) of the type of carbohydrate in a particular food is converted to blood sugar. It's about the characteristics of the carbohydrate, but not the amount.
- **The glycemic load (GL)** adjusts a food's GI value based on the amount of carbohydrate is in one serving of a particular food, on a scale of 0-60. For example, watermelon has a high GI of 72, but because there is so little digestible carbohydrate per serving, it has a low glycemic load of 4. Pasta (cooked al dente) has a low GI of 22 but a high GL of 46 (any GL above 20 is high).

Foods that are both low GI and low GL include whole fruit, lentils, most beans and most vegetables (including carrots). Many traditional diets, including diets of the Mediterranean, Middle East, Latin America, Africa and South and East Asia have a low GI and GL. It's not necessarily easy to guess a food's GI or GL from how it looks or the list of ingredients on its label.

There's the fact that how our blood-sugar levels change after we eat carbohydrate-rich foods depends on what other foods we eat with them. Mixed meals and snacks that include grains, starchy vegetables or fruit along with protein and healthful fat (protein and fat have minimal effect on blood sugar) are digested more slowly, promoting gentle fluctuations in blood sugar. The whole meal has a lower glycemic load.

For healthy blood sugar levels, nutritional balance and satisfaction, I generally recommend not eating "naked carbs." When you eat carb-rich foods, eat them with a little protein and healthy fat (toast with nut butter instead of toast with jam, for example). I'll remind you of this again in Chapter 7.

The fact that we generally eat foods together with other foods means that it's not helpful to get too obsessive about choosing low-GI foods. Another reason is that emerging research suggests that how our blood sugar responds to a food varies from person to person, possibly due to differences in the gut microbiota. That's why I'm not including a list. When you base your diet on whole or less-processed carbohydrate foods and combine them with foods that provide quality protein and healthy fats, you'll do just fine!

Your gut microbiota

WHEN IT COMES TO DISEASE RISK, are your genes your destiny? Science is increasingly suggesting otherwise. As scientists look for explanations for the roots of chronic disease as well as the connections between nutrition and health, the answer may be in your gut—and what you feed it.

Your gut—or intestines, your large intestine in particular—is home to a population of bacteria and other microbes (your gut microbiota). Think of it as a whole ecosystem living inside your body's "inner tube." The state of your gut microbiota affects more than just your digestive health: an imbalance of "good" and "bad" bacteria has been linked to chronic inflammation, obesity, chronic disease and a weakened immune system.

The gut microbiota (the critters in your gut) and microbiome (the genome, or collection of genes, that belong to those critters) is an emerging area of research, and its both possible and likely that the state of our microbiota won't be responsible for everything that we think it might be. However, research so far is helping us understand that in many ways, our gut microbiota does contribute to health—or a lack of it.

Your genes and your environment interact constantly, and your gut is the largest meeting point. On security duty is your microbiota, the collection of about 100 trillion bacteria and other microbes that live in your intestines, especially your large intestine (colon).

We inherit two genomes (a complete set of genes and DNA). The human genome has about 30,000 genes and essentially remains unchanged in our lifetime. Our microbiome contains about 150 times as many genes, but changes significantly in response to our diet and lifestyle habits. Because of this changeability, our microbiome affects whether we inherit our genetic "destiny."

The "starter" microbiota you inherited from your mother at birth was more robust if you were born vaginally than if you were born via C-section (in very simple terms, the microbiota of the birth canal are different from the microbiota found on the skin, and the species found in the birth canal are apparently what we are meant to inherit). For the first few years after birth, our immune system and microbiota develop and mature together in a mutually beneficial relationship. Your personal microbiota is as individual as you are, like a bacterial fingerprint—and it's influenced by the food you eat.

How our microbiota develops in childhood may affect our risk of weight and chronic disease later in life—and inflammation is likely the common thread.

Inflammation and your gut

One reason that the state of your intestinal ecosystem has a profound effect on your health is that one layer of cells is all that separates your immune system from the contents of your gut, and inflammation is our immune system's main weapon against foreign invaders.

A healthy, balanced gut microbiota promotes a strong immune system and lower levels of chronic inflammation. An unhealthy microbiota has been linked to weight gain, asthma, allergies, and autoimmune disorders like celiac disease, type 1 diabetes, inflammatory bowel disease and rheumatoid arthritis. Increasingly, chronic inflammation is also thought to be a root cause of cardiovascular disease, type 2 diabetes and some forms of cancer.

Our diets and our exposure to antibiotics and chemicals alter our microbiota—for better or for worse. The composition of our microbiota affects how food is broken down in our bodies and how many calories and nutrients we absorb.

Care and feeding of your microbiota

BECAUSE EVERYTHING WE EAT comes into contact with our microbiota, eating a diet high in refined, heavily processed foods can knock the microbiota out of balance. The relationship between food and the microbiota is a two-way street: The food we eat affects the composition of our microbiota, and the composition of our microbiota affects how we digest and absorb our food.

The connection between what we eat and the health of our microbiota is very complex, but a good place to start is to eat a plant-based diet with lots of fruits, vegetables, whole grains and pulses (beans and lentils). This provides an abundance of prebiotics fiber, aka food for the beneficial, health-promoting bacteria you want to have living in your gut. Then, add some probiotics, bacterial species that provide us with health benefits, from foods and/or supplements. Together, prebiotics and probiotics can help maintain the delicate balance between your intestinal environment and your immune system.

Why fiber is your friend

Your microbiota adapts to its environment, and if that environment doesn't provide the fiber it needs, your microbes will instead dine on the thin layer of mucus that protects your intestinal lining, potentially leading to a "leaky gut" and all number of health problems. So nurture a stable and diverse community of intestinal critters by offering them a fiber smorgasbord from a diet rich in vegetables, fruits, whole grains and pulses (bean and lentils). These foods are rich in prebiotic fiber, or dietary fiber that escapes digestion in the small intestine but is fermented by the types of bacteria you want to have hanging around in your colon.

While many plant foods contain fermentable, prebiotic fiber, some are richer than others.

If you aren't eating a lot of fiber-rich foods, increase your intake slowly. Some prebiotic fibers can cause flatulence (gas) if you eat too much, too soon. They can also cause significant digestive distress in some people who have irritable bowel syndrome.

Good food for your microbiota also comes from resistant starch, which is found in whole grains as well as in cooked and cooled pasta, rice and potatoes. Some people find that it's easier to boost intake of resistant starch than fiber.

Top picks for prebiotic fiber

- Almonds
- Artichokes
- Asparagus
- Bananas
- Brassicas (broccoli, Brussels sprout, cabbage)
- Burdock root
- Cereal grains such as whole wheat, barley and rye (note, these grains contain gluten, so anyone with celiac disease or gluten sensitivity will need to avoid them, obviously)
- Chicory root
- Endive
- Garlic
- Greens (especially dandelion greens)
- Jerusalem artichoke
- Jicama
- Kiwi
- Leeks
- Legumes (beans and lentils)
- Mushrooms
- Oats
- Onions
- Plantains
- Salsify

Seeding the microbial garden

The World Health Organization (WHO) defines probiotics as live microorganisms which, when administered in adequate amounts, confer a health benefit on the host. One common myth about fermented foods is that they are the same thing as probiotics. To be a probiotic food, a fermented food must retain an adequate level of live microbes that have been shown to have a health benefit. Not all fermented foods reach that bar. Some fermented foods don't retain live cultures, and those that do don't necessarily have probiotic functions. Confused yet?

Fermented foods include yogurt and kefir (fermented milk), tempeh and miso (fermented soy), kombucha (fermented tea) as well as fermented vegetables like sauerkraut, pickles and kimchi. Live micro-organisms in fermented foods are rarely defined, let alone tested for to determine if they confer probiotic health benefits. One reason may be logistical—the specific organisms in foods like kimchi, sauerkraut and miso vary by batch, manufacturer and location. In some cases, probiotic bacteria is specifically added to fermented foods like yogurt, kefir or kombucha, making these foods the "delivery vehicle" for the probiotic.

Many fermented foods contain millions of viable microbes, and many of those survive passage through the digestive tract. It's unlikely that these microbes take up permanent residence in your gut yet, they still have demonstrated health benefits. Researchers are trying to better understand what aspects of a fermented food—the live microbe, a metabolite produced during fermentation, or the nutrients in the food—contributes to any observed health benefits.

Even though live cultures are one important way fermented foods can benefit us, it's not the only way. For example, the bacteria and yeast that are used in the manufacture of sourdough bread are inactivated by the heat of baking, but during the fermentation, sourdough bacteria help break down some of the gluten—although not quite enough to be gluten-free.

Fermentation of fiber-rich foods can also make certain nutrients more bioavailable and produce new bioactive compounds that may help reduce inflammation and improve health in other ways. Take fermented dairy—it's often more digestible than non-fermented milk because microbes digest lactose and break down proteins into peptides (small protein fragments) and amino acids.

What about probiotic supplements?

Should you take probiotics in pill form? If you're healthy and not taking antibiotics, probably not, because there's little research, for now, on any general health benefits from probiotic supplements, as the focus has been on specific health conditions, such as inflammatory bowel disease. This means that the health claims often exceed the evidence. Instead, nurture the good bacteria you already have with healthy, prebiotic-containing foods and maybe give your gut health a little extra boost with fermented foods. As a bonus, these foods contribute other nutrients you need for a healthful diet.

If you have irritable bowel syndrome (IBS) or a history of antibiotic use—antibiotics, especially "broad spectrum" antibiotics, are tough on your microbiota—talk to your doctor about probiotics. If you could benefit from probiotic supplements, it's important to get one that has the bacterial strains you need. Speaking of antibiotics, let me offer this gentle reminder that it's important to only take antibiotics when you need them (and there are times when you really, really do) and not when you don't (like when you have a virus, because antibiotics kill bacteria, not viruses). Improper use of antibiotics in this country is contributing to antibiotic resistance (more and more types of bacteria are able to resist the effects of antibiotics). While overuse of antibiotics in livestock has (justifiably) received a lot of attention in recent years, we humans contribute to antibiotic resistance every time we take antibiotics when we don't really need them, or stop taking them early when we DO need them just because we "feel better."

Encourage diversity with the right fats

Diets high in saturated fat are harmful to microbiota diversity by encouraging the growth of harmful bacterial species, so opt for plant-based monounsaturated fats like olive oil, avocados, nuts and seeds. Another way to reduce saturated fat is to include more plant-based meals in your week, a la Meatless Monday.

Fueling your fermentation factory

Eating food rich in prebiotic fiber along with fermented foods promotes the growth of bacteria that break down plant starches and fibers into short-chain fatty acids (SCFAs). Some SCFAs may protect against inflammation and cancer, while others help us absorb essential minerals from our food, including calcium, magnesium and iron.

Individuals who consistently eat plant-based diets, such as vegan, vegetarian or Mediterranean diets, tend to have higher levels of SCFAs. This suggests that the amount of fermentable fiber matters more than the diet itself. Because not all fiber is the same, when you eat a variety of whole plant foods you nourish the microbes that can break down that fiber and encourage a more diverse and robust gut ecosystem overall.

The Mediterranean diet

A DELICIOUS WAY TO GET more gut-friendly plant foods into your meals is to go Mediterranean. The traditional Mediterranean diet is a time-tested plant-based diet that's rich in whole foods and very little highly processed foods. There's a huge variety of foods to choose from, and even more delicious ways to prepare these foods.

That traditional Mediterranean-style diets are an optimal way to eat isn't exactly breaking news, considering that this way of eating was "discovered" way back in the 1950s. What is news is the growing body of scientific evidence that this diet has the potential to prevent a number of the chronic diseases that can reduce our quality of life—and perhaps even shorten our lives.

So, what exactly is the Mediterranean diet? In its classic form, it's an approximation of the traditional dietary patterns of people who live in areas bordering the Mediterranean Sea. In particular, the olive-growing areas of Crete, Greece and southern Italy.

In more practical, modern terms, it's a diet that's rich in fruits, vegetables, legumes and whole grains. Fish is more common than poultry and much more common than red meat. Virgin olive oil is the primary source of fat, and moderate consumption of red wine during meals is common. It includes a serving or two a day of dairy foods (often yogurt), and olives and nuts are enjoyed several times a week. Eggs and sweets make an appearance a few times a week.

The magic of synergy

There has been a lot of research into why this way of eating tends to be associated with lower rates of heart disease and other chronic diseases. Earlier efforts focused on trying to isolate which parts of the diet were responsible for these positive effects. Was it the olive oil? The red wine? The relative lack of red meat? The abundant fruits and vegetables? More recently, a number of studies have found that the diet as a whole is greater than the sum of its parts. The reason? Synergy.

This isn't too surprising, given that we don't eat nutrients. We eat foods, which are combined into meals that in turn are combined into a complete pattern of eating that can contribute to, or detract from, our health. That's because the nutrients in our food are rarely soloists. They interact with each other. It's not about the olive oil. It's not about the red wine. It's about the whole dietary package.

Let's consider what the various voices in this dietary chorus bring to the stage. The plentiful fruits and vegetables and moderate amounts of nuts deliver a load of phytonutrients, antioxidant vitamins, fiber and other important nutrients. The virgin olive oil has the healthful qualities of the olive itself, plus significant amounts of phytonutrients that also act as antioxidants. And then there is the red wine, which provides even more antioxidants, as well as anti-inflammatory actions that may benefit heart health.

Part of the deliciousness of eating Mediterranean comes from the fact that so many countries and food cultures fall under the Mediterranean diet umbrella. The countries that border the Mediterranean Sea include not just Greece, and the southern parts of Italy, France and Spain, but also Lebanon, Turkey, Morocco and several others. It's a satisfying way to eat that also offers heart-healthy monounsaturated fatty acids, inflammation-fighting phytonutrients, gut-friendly prebiotic fiber, and a wealth of vitamins, minerals and antioxidants.

The Mediterranean diet is not low-fat. But it's the addition of healthy fats from olive oil, nuts and fish that may make this diet tastier and easier to stick with than many low-fat diets. Sautéing vegetables in olive oil and dressing salads in real vinaigrette makes vegetables more delicious and flavorful, encouraging us to eat more of them. And it's good to enjoy your veggies!

Bringing the Mediterranean home

The Mediterranean diet isn't about any one particular food—it's about how a variety of nutrient-rich foods work together. Still, it's helpful to know what foods you can include to make your diet more Mediterranean. Here are a few:

- **Greens, greens and more greens.** Dark leafy greens are rich in vitamins, minerals and phytonutrients, as well as plant-based omega 3 fatty acids. We don't have access to the more than 150 types of edible wild greens found on the Greek island of Ikaria, but we can forage for "weeds" like dandelion greens and purslane and enjoy cultivated greens like kale, beet greens, mustard greens and collard greens. Add greens to frittatas, scrambled eggs or bean and lentil soups. Sauté greens with garlic and finish with a squeeze of lemon and enjoy raw salads of dark leafy greens, dressed with an olive oil vinaigrette.
- **Pulses (beans and lentils).** Pulses are an important part of the Mediterranean diet, especially chickpeas (garbanzo beans), lentils, fava beans and other pulses are common ingredients in soups, stews and spreads (hummus), contributing protein, fiber and nutrients.
- **Herbs.** Herbs are high in antioxidant and anti-inflammatory phytonutrients. Each region in the Mediterranean has a different flavor palette, but herbs and spices are universally important in the Mediterranean cuisine. Do as they do in the Mediterranean, and add fresh herbs to salads to give then an antioxidant boost.
- **Lemons.** Lemons were brought to the Mediterranean from the Far East eons ago. The acidity and high flavonoid con-

tent of lemon juice and lemon peels may have a beneficial impact on blood sugar by slowing stomach emptying after a meal. Lemon juice is a staple ingredient in hummus, but you can also go Med by squeezing lemon juice on salads, fish, roasted broccoli, beans, into soups and drinking water.

- **Nuts.** Almonds, walnuts, pistachios, hazelnuts, and other nuts are staples in the Mediterranean diet. Eat them on their own or chop and add them to salads and other dishes for heart-healthy fats along with protein, fiber and a wealth of nutrients.

- **Olive oil.** Italy, Spain and Greece are the top three producers of olive oil in the world, and olive oil is the common dietary denominator throughout the Mediterranean. Olive oil is the principal source of dietary fat for both cooking and baking, and is important not just for its antioxidant and anti-inflammatory properties, but also because it makes it all those vegetable and pulses more delicious!

What are phytonutrients?

Phytonutrients, also called phytochemicals, are natural substances found in plant foods that have also been found to have beneficial health effects in humans. Scientists think that phytonutrients are responsible for much of the disease protection offered by diets high in fruits, vegetables, beans, whole grains, and plant-based beverages such as tea and wine.

Scientists have identified thousands of phytonutrients, but not all of them have been thoroughly studied (yet). Certain phytonutrients may be called antioxidants, flavonoids, flavanols, flavanones, isoflavones, catechins, epicatechins, anthocyanins, anthocyanidins, proanthocyanidins, isothiocyanates, carotenoids, allyl sulfides, polyphenols, phenolic acids, and many other names. You'll learn more in Chapter 5.

Anti-inflammatory diets

WHAT DOES AN ANTI-INFLAMMATORY, microbiota-nurturing diet look like?

It's made of real, whole foods! Various versions floating around, but at its core, it's a plant-based, whole foods diet rich in these healthful components:

- **Phytonutrients.** Phytonutrients are often tied to pigments (colors) and fiber in plant foods. Choose fruits and vegetables from all parts of the color spectrum ("eat the rainbow"), especially berries, tomatoes, orange and yellow fruits, and dark leafy greens. Different colors = different phytonutrients.
- **Fiber.** Up your fiber intake by eating more fruit (especially berries), vegetables (especially beans), and whole grains.
- **Vitamins and minerals.** Vitamins and minerals play essential roles in helping your cells go about their constant business of helping your body run optimally.

Primary anti-inflammatory food groups

An anti-inflammatory diet is based on whole plant foods, with smaller amounts of animal foods. It minimizes sugar and highly processed foods. It's really not as complicated as some books, articles or blogs make it out to be. Here's the foundation:

- **Vegetables and fruit.** Eating an abundance of fruits and vegetables from all parts of the color spectrum will provide you with a variety of antioxidants and health-promoting plant phytonutrients. Choose organic whenever possible to reduce exposure to pesticide residues.
- **Whole intact grains.** Choose grains that are intact (brown rice, quinoa) or in a few large pieces (bulgur, steel cut oats). For bread, think whole grain over white, dense over fluffy, naturally fermented (sourdough) over "regular" yeast fermented. If you enjoy pasta, eat it in moderation and cook it al dente (firm to the bite).
- **Pulses.** Plant-based proteins like pulses (beans, lentils and peas) and less-processed forms of soy (tofu, tempeh, edamame, soymilk) can help reduce inflammation, in part because they are fiber-rich.
- **Healthy fats (nuts, seeds, avocados, olive oil).** Use extra-virgin olive oil as your main oil. Expeller-pressed organic canola oil is another option if you want a neutral-tasting oil. Include moderate amounts of avocados, nuts and seeds in your meals or snacks, as these contain wonderful heart-

healthy, anti-inflammatory fats.

- **Fish.** For non-vegetarians, this is the best source of animal protein because of its lovely heart-healthy, anti-inflammatory omega-3 fatty acids. Wild Alaskan salmon, wild cod and sardines are top picks.
- **Other animal protein in moderation.** While it's important to get enough protein (more on this in Chapter 6), excessive amounts of meat, and to a lesser extent poultry, milk and dairy, can be inflammatory. Your best picks for an anti-inflammatory diet are omega-3 fortified eggs, quality yogurt and small amounts of natural cheese (i.e., real cheese, not processed products like so-called "American" cheese.) When purchasing animal-based proteins, go organic whenever you can. And balance them with lots of non-starchy vegetables!
- **Alcohol in moderation or not at all.** If you do choose to imbibe, red wine is preferred.

Foods to limit

I prefer to talk about foods to include rather than foods to limit, but I think when talking about what foods are anti-inflammatory, it makes sense to at least mention which foods or food components have been shown to be inflammatory:

- **Partially hydrogenated oils (aka trans fats).** This includes margarine and vegetable shortening (unless they are clearly labeled otherwise), and all products with partially hydrogenated oil in the list of ingredients.
- **Saturated fat, in excess.** You find saturated fat in full-fat dairy products (cheese, cream, butter, whole milk) as well as poultry skin, fatty meats, palm kernel oil and coconut oil. Based on current research, I'm a little less concerned about full-fat plain yogurt and quality cheese (which is why I gave them a thumbs up above under "other animal protein in moderation"). Even though they don't deserve their health halos, I think coconut oil and grass-fed butter are OK in moderation, from a culinary standpoint.
- **Sugar and white flour in excess.** I'm not in favor of completely shunning sugar and white flour, because these ingredients are found in many foods that can bring real joy and pleasure. But they are also found in a lot of foods that offer no nutrition and honestly aren't all that delicious if you really pay attention to them while you're eating them (read:

packaged cookies and snack foods, cheap baked goods, fast food burger buns). When these foods regularly find their way into your meals and snacks, they do have the potential to make you feel less than your best, and todo some harm.

When you make a point to reduce heavily processed foods, not only are you avoiding refined white flour and sugar, but you are avoiding partially hydrogenated oils and low-quality, damaged fats that promote inflammation.

General tips:

- Aim for variety.
- Include as much fresh food as possible.
- Limit processed foods and fast food to occasional indulgences.
- Eat an abundance of fresh fruits and vegetables.
- When availability and budget allow, choose organic foods.

Anti-inflammatory powerhouses

WHILE VIRTUALLY ANY FOOD from the anti-inflammatory diet food categories discussed above can contribute to preventing or lowering chronic inflammation and promoting optimal health and well-being, here are some anti-inflammatory superstars worth knowing about.

- **Cruciferous family.** Vegetables from the cruciferous family—broccoli, cabbage, Brussels sprouts, kale and cauliflower—are especially rich in antioxidants and inflammation-fighting and anti-cancer phytonutrients. The most notable phytonutrient group in this veggie family are the isothiocyanates, a group of sulfur-containing compounds that gives cruciferous veggies their sharp taste. Think of wasabi, mustard, watercress, broccoli and so on. Try to eat veggies from this family daily!
- **Allium family.** If you love garlic, enjoy it daily. Other members of the allium family (onions, leeks, shallots) are other flavorful additions to the anti-inflammatory diet, but garlic reigns supreme.
- **Green tea.** All types of true tea—green, oolong and black—contain inflammation-fighting phytonutrients, but green is the top choice, as it is especially rich in the anti-inflammatory, anti-cancer flavanol (a type of phytonutrient), epigal-

locatechin gallate, or EGCG. Japanese green tea, matcha in particular, has higher levels of EGCG. Herbal teas don't have the same benefit, because they aren't true teas (i.e., they don't come from the leaves of the Camellia sinensis bush). What about coffee? Coffee does contain phytonutrients, but in excess it can contribute to inflammation, due to the caffeine.

- **Spices.** Spices are more than just flavoring agents—they are also packed with phytonutrients (more on this in Chapter 8). Ginger, turmeric and cinnamon are particularly noted for their anti-inflammatory properties.

Putting these foods to use

What if you, well, hate, some of the foods on the powerhouse list? I encourage you to give them another try. Take green tea for example…lots of people love green tea, but many people don't. First, there are many types of green tea, and it may take some experimenting to find one you like. Second, different types of green tea have different recommended brewing times…if you've had green tea that's brewed for too long, that may account for your dislike. Give it another go!

As for the cruciferous family, if you hate kale but love broccoli or cabbage, don't sweat it. If all the veggies in that family taste to strong to you, you may be a "supertaster." I know some supertasters who have come to enjoy broccoli and Brussels sprouts by roasting them (my personal favorite) and giving themselves time for their taste buds to adjust.

Food allergies, intolerances and sensitivities

IF YOU HAVE A DIAGNOSED food allergy, intolerance or sensitivity, part of your anti-inflammatory diet includes avoiding those foods! If you eat foods that cause inflammation in your intestines or elsewhere in your body, that can lead to chronic inflammation. Some conditions that are aggravated by certain foods include:

- Food allergies
- Celiac disease
- Non-celiac gluten sensitivity
- Inflammatory bowel disease (Crohn's disease and colitis)
- Irritable bowel syndrome
- Lactose intolerance
- Other food intolerances and sensitivities

Don't assume that you need to avoid gluten, dairy products or commonly allergenic foods if you don't have an established problem with them. That said, if you suspect you have a food allergy or sensitivity, seek medical advice so you can get a correct diagnosis. Some health conditions with symptoms that seem food-related are more serious than others—don't try to self-diagnose!

Chapter summary

Are you getting a clearer picture about why your food choices can play such a big role in health? We often think about vitamins, minerals, calories, protein, carbs and fat, but as we learn more about phytonutrients and the critters the live in our gut, things just get more and more interesting!

Here are the main takeaways from Chapter 4:

- Inflammation can help us or hurt us.
- The Glycemic Index isn't gospel.
- It pays off to nurture your gut microbiota with good food.
- As an eating roadmap for both pleasure and health, it's hard to go wrong with the Mediterranean diet.
- Why an anti-inflammatory diet is simply a healthy diet (no weird food restrictions needed).
- Who needs to be concerned about food allergies, intolerances and sensitivities.

Coming up in Chapter 5, The Power of Produce:

- Fruits and vegetables
- Organic vs. Non-organic
- Eating seasonally
- Fresh vs. Frozen
- Phytonutrients
- The joys of dark leafy greens

The Power of Produce

IN CASE YOU STILL NEED CONVINCING after the last chapter, I'll rhapsodize over the many virtues of loading up on produce. While we can't live on vegetables and fruits alone, they are vital to good health (plus they make for a pretty plate, with their widely varying color and texture).

In this chapter, I'll talk about:

- The low-down on **fruits and vegetables**, and why they play different yet slightly overlapping roles in a healthful, nutritious diet.
- How to put the **organic vs. non-organic** debate into perspective, so you can feel more confident about your shopping decisions.
- **Eating seasonally**...Does it matter? Does it limit you to eating kale and root vegetable in the winter? Let's discuss.
- Why vegetables and fruits are so darn good for you. Vitamins? Sure. Minerals? Sure. But mostly, it's about the **phytonutrients**.
- Cue the orchestra, because I'll wrap up this chapter with a serenade to the joys of **dark leafy greens**.

Fruits and vegetables

IN CHAPTER 3, I talked about the power of plant-based diets. In Chapter 4, I talked about anti-inflammatory diets and Mediterranean-style diets. The foundation of all of those styles of eating is vegetables and (to a slightly lesser degree) fruits. Why? Because vegetables are crucial to health or vitality...the Latin word for vegetables even means "to enliven or animate."

Although we can't live on vegetables and fruits alone (not enough protein and fat), they are absolute nutrient powerhouses. While you store some nutrients in your cells and tissues, most micronutrients (vitamins and minerals) can't be stored. That means you need to get them in your diet every day. Vegetables provide an amazing array of vitamins, minerals, phytonutrients and fiber as well as modest amounts of protein and essential fats.

Non-starchy vegetables

Non-starchy vegetables are extremely nutrient-rich, which means that they pack in maximum nutrients with minimum calories. This is good news when you want to improve your health and be a weight that's healthy for you. Because they are high in water, vitamins, minerals and phytonutrients and low in protein and fat, non-starchy vegetables are the perfect complement to more concentrated sources of carbohydrates, fat and protein, such as whole grains, beans, meat, poultry, eggs and dairy foods.

So what's better for nutrition: raw or cooked? While many nutrients are partially lost when you cook them in water, the fiber and the basic nutrient profile remains. Another fact to consider is that your body absorbs some nutrients better from cooked vegetables. So it's a bit of a wash, really. To make the most of the bounty of nutrients in your veggies, include both raw and cooked in your diet. If you want to minimize nutrient loss when you cook your veg, roast them or cook them briefly (until crisp-tender) in water or steam.

Vegetables tend to get relegated to lunch, dinner and the occasional snack while fruit reigns supreme at breakfast. When you are trying to eat more vegetables, you can increase how often you eat them, how much you eat when you do eat them, or both. Why not sneak some into breakfast? The two ways I like to do this is by cooking dark leafy greens and other veggies with scrambled eggs, or adding greens to my smoothies. On the following page is a basic list of non-starchy veggies:

Arugula	Ginger root
Artichoke	Green beans
Asparagus	Jalapeno peppers
Bean sprouts	Kale
Beet greens	Lettuces
Beets	Mushrooms
Bell peppers (any color)	Mustard greens
Broccoli	Onions
Brussels sprouts	Parsley
Cabbage	Radishes
Carrots	Radicchio
Cauliflower	Snap beans
Celery	Snow peas
Chives	Shallots
Collard greens	Spinach
Cucumber	Summer squash
Dandelion greens	Swiss chard
Eggplant	Tomatoes
Endive	Turnip greens
Fennel	Watercress
Garlic	Zucchini

Starchy vegetables

Starchy vegetables are rich in high-quality carbohydrates as well as vitamins, minerals, antioxidants, phytonutrients and fiber. The main difference between starchy and non-starchy vegetables is that starchy veggies are higher in calories and provide about 15 grams of carbohydrates per serving, while non-starchy vegetables have about 5 grams. You also need to cook most starchy vegetables before you eat them.

Example of starchy vegetables include potatoes, sweet potatoes, winter squash, plantains, corn and peas. When planning your meals, treat starchy vegetables the same way you would treat grain foods, because the amount of carbohydrate is similar. While starchy vegetables are wonderfully nutritious, they won't make up for a lack of broccoli, leafy greens and other non-starchy veggies.

Fruit

Fruit is considered one of nature's perfect foods. It's natural and healthy. It's juicy, with a high water content (like the human body itself!). It's a wonderful source of vitamins, minerals and phytonutrients. Yes, fruit is high in natural sugar, but it's sugar in a fiber-rich, nutrient-rich package. Whole fruit is the most natural, nutritious way to get that sweet taste we're born to love.

Avocados and olives are technically fruits, too, but for nutrition purposes we include them in the healthy fats category.

Organic vs. non-organic

THE HEALTH VALUE OF ORGANIC FOOD is a frequent talking point—and even fighting point—in the media. The debate heated up in the aftermath of a large research study published a few years ago suggesting that organic produce and meat is no more nutritious than non-organic, "conventional" food.

You might wonder, are organic foods really healthier foods? Or, is this just another example of a food belief system, as in "I believe this food is healthier, so therefore it is…never mind what science says"?

The study in question, conducted by Stanford University, has been picked apart endlessly. One criticism is that the type of study, a meta-analysis (a statistical compilation of numerous research studies done by other people), may not be suitable for something as variable as agriculture. Everything from weather, geography, plant variety and degree of ripeness when picked can affect nutrient levels in produce.

Can we say conclusively that organic produce is more nutritious? Maybe not. Maybe never. But food scientists and plant biologists know of at least a few ways that organically grown fruits and vegetables can develop more nutrients. For example, without the protection of chemical pesticides, plants need to beef up their innate defenses by producing phytonutrients. Conveniently, these natural compounds are repellent to pests but health-promoting when eaten by humans.

Let's identify the real issue

If we're worried about getting enough nutrition from our fruits and vegetables, there is a bigger issue at hand: Most people are simply not eating enough fruits and vegetables. Market research data tells us that, on average, children and adults eat slightly more than one cup of vegetables and half a cup of fruit each day. That's a far cry from the MyPlate recommendations to "make half your plate fruits and vegetables."

If nutrients are important to you, also consider how far your apples or tomatoes travel to get to your plate. The shorter the time and distance from harvest to table, the fresher and more nutritious your fruits and veggies. Produce is often picked unripe for long-distance shipping, before it has had a chance to reach it full nutrient potential. Shipping and storage conditions can further degrade nutrients.

Are organics right for you?

Nutrition aside, are there reasons to buy organic? I think so. Eating organic foods reduces your exposure to chemical fertilizers and pesticides. Supporting organic farming reduces the exposure of farmworkers—and the environment—to these chemicals. Livestock raised under organic guidelines aren't fed antibiotics or growth hormones. Finally, organic farming generally goes hand-in-hand with good land stewardship.

Keep in mind that locally grown produce, even when conventional, needs less chemical processing since it doesn't need to be shipped. So go pay a visit to your nearest farmer's market!

Eating seasonally

ONCE UPON A TIME, eating seasonally wasn't a lifestyle choice—it was the only choice. You ate what grew in your own backyard or on nearby farms, then you "put up" some of the harvest's bounty to get you through the winter. If you lived in a northern climate, enjoying something as simple as a California or Florida orange in the winter was a luxury.

Today, boundless growth in domestic and global transportation means you can eat cantaloupes from Chile while Eastern Washington melon farms lie under a blanket of snow. You can partake of produce that doesn't even grow in North America, such as bananas, pineapples, mangos—and coffee. Is that a good thing, or would we be better off returning to our seasonal roots?

With the evolution of the locavore movement, eating seasonally and eating locally have become almost synonymous. While there is no scientific research specifically linking improved health to eating seasonally within your own climate, there are certain benefits to favoring locally grown foods, in season.

Better nutrition. Buying local, in-season produce when you can means your produce is fresher and most likely more nutritious, because it hasn't traveled terribly far to reach your kitchen. Produce destined for shipping may be picked before it fully ripened, preventing it from developing a complete array of vitamins, minerals and phytonutrients. Nutrients degrade even further when exposed to the light, heat and air that are typical of transport and storage.

Lower cost. When produce is in season locally, prices generally drop, especially at the peak of harvest when supplies are abundant. "Off-season" imported produce can be comparatively more expensive due of shipping costs. Purchase what's growing in your area now and reap the financial rewards.

Fuller flavor. Let's face it, fresh summer strawberries and tomatoes taste far better than their winter cardboard counterparts. Fruits and vegetables lose more than nutrients with shipping and storage—they lose flavor and moisture, too. Fresh, local produce has fuller flavor and better texture, helping you build memorable taste experiences that you can look forward to each year with the changing of the seasons.

More satisfaction. Eating seasonally may suit our bodies. Fresh green salads and juicy peaches help keep us cool and hydrated in the warm months, while cooked greens and soups and stews chock full of carrots, beans, potatoes and parsnips help warm us when we come inside from the chill and the rain.

The Art of Compromise

It's easy to eat seasonally with a lot of variety in the summer months, but staying seasonal in some areas of the country gets a little more hardcore come winter, no matter how much you enjoy hearty greens and root vegetables. How do you still have the variety you may crave while following some semblance of a seasonal ideal?

Go almost local. Choose produce grown in California or other warmer-winter states rather than specimens grown in South America, Africa, Australia or New Zealand.

Buy frozen. Frozen berries and other produce are picked at the peak of ripeness and immediately sent for processing, preserving most of their flavor and nutrition.

Prioritize. Maybe you can't live without fresh green salads in December—or without coffee anytime—but you're content to wait until summer to have corn, peaches and tomatoes.

Beyond vitamins and minerals: phytonutrients

THE TERM PHYTOCHEMICALS refers to a wide variety of compounds produced by plants, and usually is used to refer only to those compounds that may affect health (in this case, they are often referred to as phytonutrients). Phytonutrients are found in vegetables, fruits, beans, grains and other plants.

Each phytonutrient is found in many different plant sources and has slightly different proposed health benefits. While they are not essential nutrients, in the way that vitamins and minerals are, they are believed to be one of the reasons for the health benefits of diets rich in fruits, vegetables, legumes, whole grains and nuts. However, evidence that these effects are due to specific nutrients or phytonutrients is currently limited.

Because plant-based foods are complex mixtures of bioactive compounds, including vitamins, minerals, phytonutrients and fiber, it's difficult to tease apart the potential health effects of individual phytonutrients from the health effects of the foods that contain those phytonutrients. In other words, it's thought that phytonutrients, vitamins, minerals and fiber, all present in fruits and vegetables, work together in whole plant foods to promote good health and lower disease risk. This means that putting phytonutrients into a pill won't confer the same benefits as eating the phytonutrient in its natural whole food packaging.

What are the phytonutrients in food?

Some researchers estimate that there are as many as 4,000 phytonutrients. Indeed, thousands have been identified, although only a small portion of those have been studied closely. These include:

Anthocyanidins: Responsible for the gorgeous red, purple and blue colors in berries. May help keep your blood vessels healthy. Food sources include blueberries, blackberries, plums, cranberries, raspberries, red onions, red potatoes, red radishes and strawberries.

Carotenoids (including beta-carotene): Found in orange fruits and vegetables and dark, leafy green veggies. May benefit the immune system, vision, skin health and bone health. Food sources include pumpkin, sweet potato, carrots, winter squash, cantaloupe, apricots, spinach, collard greens, kale and broccoli

Catechin and the epicatechins: These phytonutrients are associated with a lower risk of heart disease and certain cancers, in part because of their proposed anti-inflammatory properties. Food sources include tea, red wine, cocoa powder, dark chocolate, grapes, plums and beans.

Indoles and isothiocyanates: The reason that cruciferous vegetables are phytonutrient powerhouses. Believed to have inflammation- and cancer-fighting properties. Food sources include broccoli, Brussels sprouts, cabbage, kale and cauliflower.

Isoflavones: Found in soybeans. Possible benefits include easing of menopausal symptoms, breast cancer prevention, bone health, reduction of joint inflammation and lower cholesterol. These benefits have been studied in whole soy products (for example, tofu, tempeh, edamame, miso, soymilk) but not in the isolated soy protein found in many powders and protein bars.

Lutein: Found in many green vegetables. May have benefits for eye health, heart health and cancer prevention. Food sources include collard greens, kale, spinach, broccoli, Brussels sprouts, lettuces and artichokes.

Lycopene: Found in red and pink fruits and vegetables. May help prevent prostate cancer and promote heart health. The heating process makes it easier for your body to absorb lycopene (which is why ketchup and tomato paste are better sources than fresh tomatoes). Food sources include tomatoes, pink grapefruit, red peppers, watermelon, pomegranates and tomato products.

Organosulfur compounds: The reason that the allium (onion) family of vegetables are phytonutrient powerhouses. Believed to have powerful anti-inflammatory and anti-cancer properties. Found in garlic (best source), onions, leeks, shallots, scallions and chives.

Proanthocyanidins: This group of phytonutrients has strong antioxidant properties, and may help reduce the risk of heart disease and cancer. The proanthocyanidins in cranberries may help protect against urinary tract infections. Food sources include tea, cocoa, many berries, grapes and grape juice, cranberries and cranberry juice, and red wine.

Resveratrol: One of the reasons for the suggested health benefits of moderate red wine consumption. May promote heart and lung health, reduce inflammation and help prevent cancer. Food sources include red wine, peanuts, grape skin and grape juice.

That's far from a comprehensive list. A few other notables include curcumin (turmeric and mustard), vanillin (vanilla), caffeic acid and chlorogenic acid (coffee), cinnamic acid (cinnamon and aloe), capsaicin (chili peppers) and a whole collection of phytonutrients are found in olive oil.

The joys of dark leafy greens

I HOPE THAT THE LINGERING infatuation with kale is more than a passing fancy, because kale is not only awesome, it's awesomely good for you.

Let me be blunt: kale is a nutritional superstar. It's a dark, leafy green, but it's also a cruciferous vegetable. That means it's the best of two nutrient-packed worlds. It is loaded with antioxidant vitamins, as are most dark leafy greens, but it's also rich in the phytonutrients that are a hallmark among the Cruciferae. As I just covered, phytonutrients have been shown to have a protective effect against inflammation and certain types of cancer.

How can you prepare kale? Let me count the ways. You can braise it, sauté it, stir-fry it or bake it into kale chips. You can add it to soups, omelets, casseroles and other baked dishes. Raw, you can blend it into smoothies or eat it as a salad green. (One tip: Unless you're using baby kale, it's often easier to massage oil into the leaves than to simply toss it like you would a salad with tender greens.)

While kale is a superstar, it's not the only star. There's a whole wonderful world of dark leafy greens out there, which is great news, because some people will just never like kale (and that's OK). Here's a short list of the heavy hitters:

- **Dandelion greens** are one of the top four green vegetables for overall nutritional value, according to the U.S. Department of Agriculture. They contain more beta-carotene than any other green veggie, and have more vitamin A than any food except cod liver oil and beef liver! They are also rich in calcium, potassium, vitamin K and fiber. My favorite way to enjoy them is to trim off the tougher bottom stem and toss the leaves in a warm vinaigrette. This balances out their slight bitterness and tenderizes them a bit.
- **Spinach** nips at kale's heels in terms of nutritional excellence. It's one of the best food sources of vitamin K, which is important for bone health. It's also rich in flavonoids, phytonutrients that do double duty as antioxidants and cancer-fighters.
- **Swiss chard** is a close relative of spinach—and of beets—that is not only beautiful, but is a great source of beta-carotene, vitamin A, potassium, calcium and vitamin C. You can cook the stems with the leaves, or treat them as two separate vegetables. Much like spinach, the leaves cook quickly.
- **Collard greens** are a good source of magnesium, potassium and vitamins A, C and K. Plus, one cup of cooked collards has as much calcium as 8 ounces of milk, with 5 grams of fiber to boot. Collards are a thick, hearty green (even more so than kale), which means they benefit from cooking. My favorite way to prepare them is to tear them into pieces, steam them in a covered pot with about a half-inch of water until they wilt, then uncover the pot and move them around with tongs as they continue cooking and the water evapo-

rates. I finish them off with a touch of maple syrup and hot sauce (usually Sriracha, sometimes Tabasco) and freshly ground salt and pepper.

Dark leafy greens are so good for you and so versatile, I encourage you to experiment. If you have even a hint of a green thumb, you can even grow them yourself. They're as beautiful in the garden as they are nutritious and delicious on the plate.

Chapter summary

After reading this chapter, I'm sure that if you had any lingering doubts about why it's great to "eat your veggies," that they've been swept away! While you can't live on vegetables alone (as you'll see in the next chapter), I hope that you look at how you're doing on the vegetable front and bump up your intake if you need to.

Here are the main takeaways from Chapter 5:

- Vegetables and fruits are the foundation of both the Mediterranean diet and anti-inflammatory diets.
- When considering organic vs. non-organic foods, nutrition may not be the deciding factor.
- However, eating seasonally is one way to increase the nutritional value of your produce.
- Phytonutrients, with their anti-inflammatory, anti-oxidant and even anti-cancer properties, are likely one of the major reasons that vegetables and fruits are so good for us.
- While kale is rightfully a nutritional superstar, there are many nutritious and delicious ways to celebrate the joys of dark leafy greens.

Coming up in Chapter 6, Staying Strong:

- Protein and your body
- The power of plant protein
- Myths about protein
- Why exercise?
- The 3-legged stool of fitness
- Fitting in exercise

Staying Strong

POPEYE MAY HAVE gained his strength from spinach, but we can't live on vegetables alone. If you want to be strong and feel strong, you need muscle. As we pass out of younger adulthood, we lose lean muscle unless we take action to stop that loss. The two main muscle-preserving tools in your toolbox are eating adequate protein and exercising regularly. Use it or lose it!

In this chapter, I'll talk about:

- **Protein and your body,** or how much and how often you need it.
- **The power of plant proteins,** whether or not you also choose to eat meat, poultry, fish, eggs or dairy.
- **Myths about protein** (because you know I love to myth-bust).
- **Why exercise?** Hint, there are a million good reasons.
- **The 3-legged stool of fitness,** because balance is everything (and I don't just mean being able to stand on one foot).
- **Fitting in exercise** in a day filled with other demands on your time. Yes, you can do it.

Protein and your body

EATING ADEQUATE PROTEIN is important for everybody, no matter what gender you are, how old you are or how healthy you are—although those factors each play a role in your individual needs. Your body needs protein to build and maintain lean muscle, to recover from illness or injury, to support a healthy immune system, and so on.

What is protein?

Proteins are made of building blocks called amino acids. Your body takes the protein from your food, disassembles it into amino acids for the "amino acid pool," then pulls amino acids from the pool to build the specific proteins you need, such as muscle fibers, blood cells, hormones and enzymes. Protein makes life possible! There are millions of proteins, and each one is unique in which amino acids it contains and how they are arranged.

There are nine essential amino acids and 11 non-essential amino acids. Essential amino acids are essential because your body can't manufacture them, so you have to get them from food. You don't have to get non-essential amino acids from your food, because your body can make them from scratch or convert them from another amino acid.

Some non-essential amino acids can become essential in certain people. For example people with the rare inherited disorder phenylketonuria (PKU) can't convert the essential amino acid phenylalanine into the non-essential amino acid tyrosine, so tyrosine becomes essential (they also have to be careful not to get too much phenylalanine, because it can build up to dangerous levels in their bodies). A less extreme example is during recovery from illness or injury, when your body's needs for the non-essential amino acids may be greater than its ability to create or convert them—so you'll need to make up the difference with food. This is one reason that our protein needs are higher when we are sick or injured.

Why do we need protein?

Proteins are found all throughout your body. About 40 percent of the proteins in your body are in your muscles, about 25 percent are in your organs (heart, liver, kidneys, etc.) and most of the rest are found in your blood and skin. Here's a little rundown of some of the important things proteins do in your body:

- **Enzymes:** These affect the rate of chemical reactions in your body.
- **Hormones:** These chemical messengers regulate metabolic

processes in your body.

- **Immune system:** Antibodies and other immune system cells are made of proteins.
- **Transport proteins:** These proteins move nutrients in and out of your cells, move other nutrients through your blood (iron, copper, vitamin A, calcium, zinc, vitamin B6) and transport cholesterol and fats in your blood (lipoproteins).
- **Buffers:** Proteins help regulate your body's acid-alkaline balance, or pH, because various amino acids can act as acids or bases (alkaline agents).

When do we need MORE protein?

I already mentioned that your protein needs increase when you are sick or injured. Protein needs also increase during times of rapid growth, including fetal growth during pregnancy, because the body needs to build more protein to make muscles, organs, blood cells, etc.

The Recommended Daily Allowance (RDA) for protein, as set by the Institute of Medicine, is 0.36 grams of protein per pound of body weight per day. This is what that would look like:

150 pounds = 54 grams per day
200 pounds = 72 grams per day
250 pounds = 90 grams per day

There are a few potential problems with this number, however. First, it's based on studies done primarily on younger adults (and not everyone is a younger adult). Second, it's based on simply replacing the protein the body loses each day (from excreted cells, enzymes, skin cell shedding, etc.). In other words, the number doesn't apply to all people, and it doesn't account for people who are sick or injured or who are trying to build lean muscle.

We lose about 1 percent of our muscle each year after age 30, unless we actively take steps to not lose it. To preserve muscle and stay healthy longer, we may need 0.5 grams of protein per pound of body weight per day. Some large observational studies have found that eating this much protein was associated with decreased risk of frailty with age. This is what 0.5g/pound/day would look like:

150 pounds = 75 grams per day
200 pounds = 100 grams per day
250 pounds = 125 grams per day

Why timing matters: optimizing intake

We are constantly making and breaking down muscle. We break down more muscle between meals, and make more muscle right after meals. The reason we tend to lose muscle with age is that older adults may not make enough muscle after meals to compensate for the amount they break down between meals. This results in loss of muscle over time.

There's been some very good research in the last several years about how our bodies use the protein we eat. One study fed 11 older adults and eight younger adults 15 grams of protein. That's roughly the amount in two ounces of meat, chicken or fish, or six ounces of Greek yogurt. Over the next 3.5 hours, the older adults incorporated fewer of the amino acids into their muscles. When the experiment was repeated, and the participants were fed more than 15 grams, the difference between the younger and older adults seemed to go away. The sweet spot for getting lots of amino acids into the muscles? About 20-30 grams per meal.

So what happens when we fall short of that per-meal goal? What happens when we go overboard? Another fascinating study fed participants, who ranged in age from 25 to 55 years, 90 grams of protein over the course of a day, in two phases:

Phase 1
Low-protein breakfast (11 grams)
Low-protein lunch (16 grams)
Protein-heavy dinner (63 grams)

Phase 2
Breakfast (30 grams)
Lunch (30 grams)
Dinner (30 grams)

They measured how much muscle the participants' bodies made during each phase. It was 25 percent higher during Phase 2 when protein was spread evenly through the day! Another study by the same researcher found that people make the same amount of protein after eating 90 grams of protein at a single meal that they do after eating 30 grams of protein. .

The power of plant proteins

BECAUSE PROTEIN HELPS BUILD MUSCLE, you might assume that animal foods like meat, poultry and fish, along with eggs and dairy, are the best sources of protein. In fact, there are many health reasons for letting plants meet more of your protein needs.

Protein: complete vs. incomplete

First, let me address a common concern about plant proteins: that they are not complete proteins. That is, they don't contain all nine of the essential amino acids.

Animal foods—meat, poultry, fish, eggs, dairy—are sources of complete protein. A few plant foods—soy and quinoa—do contain complete protein, but most plant foods, including beans, grains, nuts, vegetables and fruits, are missing one or two amino acids, or simply don't contain them in the optimal proportions for your body. We digest about 90-99 percent of the protein found in animal foods, and about 70-90 percent of the protein in plant foods (split peas are at about 70 percent, soy at about 90 percent).

The good news is that you don't need to get all of your essential amino acids from the same food. If you eat a variety of whole or minimally processed protein-rich plant foods, you will get all the amino acids you need because different sources of incomplete proteins can combine to become complementary proteins. You don't need to combine complementary proteins in the same meal as long as you get them in the course of a day.

Two classic examples of complementary protein pairings are legumes (beans, peas, lentils) with grains, and legumes with nuts or seeds. These pairings work because legumes are good sources of the amino acid lysine but are low in tryptophan and the sulfur-containing amino acids. Grains, nuts and seeds, however, are typically low in lysine but contain a good amount of tryptophan and the sulfur-containing amino acids.

Health benefits of plant proteins

It's easier than you might think to meet your protein needs from plant foods. As an added bonus, protein-rich plant foods come "packaged" with extra health-boosting features like fiber, healthy fats and a host of vitamins, minerals and phytonutrients. Animal proteins don't contain fiber or phytonutrients, and may contain unhealthy fats.

People who eat vegetarian or flexitarian (semi-vegetarian) diets tend to get more dietary fiber, magnesium, potassium, vitamins C and E, folate and phytonutrients, a diverse group of bioactive compounds found in plants that have antioxidant, anti-inflammatory and anti-cancer properties. Eating more plant protein and less animal protein is associated with a reduced risk of ovulation-related female infertility, according to research from Harvard University. Eating a plant-based diet can also lower the risk of a number of chronic diseases, including heart disease, high blood pressure and type 2 diabetes.

Does this mean you should give up meat?

More good news: you can eat and enjoy a plant-based diet even if you like eating meat (or feel better when you do). A health-promoting plant-based diet is rich in vegetables, legumes, fruits, whole grains, nuts and seeds. It can also include moderate amounts of lean meats, poultry, fish, seafood, eggs and dairy. If you choose to consume animal protein, fish and poultry are the best choices, according the Harvard School of Public Health. Many flexitarians choose to eat some fish simply for the healthy omega-3 fats.

The American Institute for Cancer Research recommends that when you do eat animal foods, try to make at least two-thirds of your plate is covered with plant foods. Another great way to tip your protein balance in favor of plant proteins is to go meatless a few days a week, a la Meatless Monday. Some ideas are to include legumes on salads and in soups and casseroles. Instead of snacking on chips or crackers and cheese, dip vegetables into a tasty bean-based dip (such as hummus) or have a piece of fresh fruit with a few nuts.

Top sources of plant proteins

Overall, beans, nuts, seeds and soy foods are the most protein-rich plant foods. Grains and vegetables contain smaller amounts of protein, but this can add up quickly when you make plants the foundation of your meals. As you fewer animal foods and more plant foods, make sure that you choose enough of the protein-rich plants. Here's the protein content of some common plant foods:

- Almonds (1 ounce): 6 grams
- Amaranth, cooked (1/2 cup): 5 grams
- Black beans, cooked (1/2 cup) 8 grams
- Chia seeds (1 ounce): 4 grams
- Chickpeas (1/2 cup): 8 grams
- Flaxseeds (1 ounce): 5 grams
- Green peas, cooked (1/2 cup): 5 grams
- Lentils, cooked (1/2 cup): 9 grams
- Peanut butter (2 tablespoons): 8 grams
- Pinto beans, cooked (1/2 cup): 8 grams
- Quinoa, cooked (1/2 cup): 4 grams
- Soymilk, unsweetened (1 cup): 7 grams
- Spinach, cooked (1/2 cup): 3 grams
- Tofu, regular (1/2 cup): 10 grams
- Walnuts (1 ounce): 4 grams

- Wheat, cooked (1/2 cup): 6 grams
- Wild rice, cooked (1/2 cup): 4 grams

Myths about protein

I LOVE BUSTING NUTRITION MYTHS, and there are a few doozies that have been kicking around about protein for what seems like forever. Thanks to the continual marching on of scientific research, we know more about how protein operates in the body, so some of what we once thought was true (based on available knowledge) we now know is not true. Trouble is, not everyone keeps up with this research, so myths persist.

Myth 1: We already get enough protein.

Fact 1: This appears true when you look at the average protein consumption in our country, and in many other countries. However, this is not true for many individuals. Why, because an average is just that—an average. This means that some people get too much protein, others get too little, and others are like Goldilocks—they're just right.

Myth 2: Too much protein is hard on your kidneys.

Fact 2: This may be true if you already have kidney disease, uncontrolled diabetes or certain other chronic health conditions that put strain on the kidneys. However, this is not true for most people, and some large, well-constructed scientific research studies have confirmed it

Myth 3: Too much protein leaches calcium from bones.

Fact 3: This myth is based on the old observation that when you eat more protein, you excrete more calcium in your urine. However, what we now know is that protein increases both the amount of calcium you excrete AND the amount of calcium you absorb from your food. In other words, you aren't losing calcium. Also research has shown that diets higher in protein may promote improved bone mass and reduced fracture risk in older adults.

Why exercise?

HEALTH AND FITNESS is not an all-or-nothing deal. It's a continuum. Your overall health, and your level of fitness, sits somewhere on a scale of 1 to 10 right at this moment. A 1 might be someone battling a terminal illness, a 2 might be someone who is struggling with multiple chronic health conditions, like high blood pressure, diabetes, high cholesterol, obesity. A 10 would be someone who is strong and flexible with great endurance, has loads of energy, a positive outlook, strong social connections, a nutrient-rich diet, and parents and grandparents who lived long, healthy lives (in other words, they have been dealt an excellent genetic hand). A 10 is not something that everyone can or should aspire to.

Your number on the continuum is based on your age, genetics, health history, socioeconomic status and past, current and future lifestyle choices. We can't control any of that...except our future choices.

Every choice you make will nudge you one direction or another on the continuum. That's why you shouldn't just throw in the towel because you've "ruined" your day sleeping in instead of going for a walk. It's also why you shouldn't put off making healthy changes until you reach some magical point in your life when you have the time/money/lack of stress to "really focus" on your health.

Maybe you don't have the internal or external resources to make big, sweeping changes, but you can do something. Small steps really do add up. Thing progress, not perfection.

Finding the joy of movement

I view getting regular physical activity the same way I view drinking enough water and eating lots of vegetables: It's good for me, but, more importantly, I don't feel good when I don't do these things. I don't train for a sport, but my daily exercise trains me for the life I want to lead. Because I make a point of maintaining a certain level of endurance, strength, balance and flexibility, the rest of my days feel easier. Gardening, cleaning out the basement, hauling groceries, carrying a heavy book bag, walking to and from mass transit. All easier. And I know that when we go on sightseeing vacations, I can walk and walk for miles if I want. That makes me happy.

What was not making me happy a few years ago was lifting weights. I've lifted weights since I was in high school, and I've always enjoyed it. I often love it. I've followed all types of lifting programs over the years, changing things up as my goals changed or as boredom crept in. So when I realized that not only was I not enjoying lifting weights, I was actually starting to feel bitter and resentful whenever it was "weight lifting day," I had to take a serious step back and reassess.

What I realized was, no matter how great weight lifting is by objective measures, if it was making me unhappy then it was not great for me... because physical activity should be enjoyable. I asked myself what would make me happy. Yoga and dance and long walks were the answers. So I turned my back on my basement weight room and embraced the yoga mat...and was much, much happier.

Because I gave myself permission to do the type of physical activity that felt right to me, instead of burying myself under "I shoulds" or "I have tos," I happily returned to my barbells and dumbbells a few weeks later…because I started missing them.

I met someone several years ago who said that a fact she has come to know and accept about herself is that, with any type of exercise, the breaking point where enjoyment ends and boredom sets in is about six weeks. When it happens, she tries something new. A new fitness adventure!

Exercise shouldn't feel like a burden. There are so many different ways to move our bodies, and we should be able to feel the benefits while we're actually moving them. Good health is about more than just physical health. It's also about mental health. And if you sacrifice mental health by gritting your teeth and doing exercise you don't like in the name of physical health, exactly how healthy are you, really?

Don't be afraid to branch out and try new things, but don't feel that you can't just stay the course if that course has made you happy and healthy. Also, if you give full effort (be honest, here) and a little bit of time to a new eating or exercise plan, but you just don't like the results you're getting, don't consider yourself a failure. There are many paths…one of them is right for you.

Motivation to move

I like to exercise. I like how I feel while exercising, and I like what it does for my health and overall wellbeing. Of course, liking something doesn't guarantee doing it. (There were an awful lot of years when I did not exercise much, and not for lack of physical activity options that I enjoyed.) The problem is, I like a lot of things. I like to garden. I like to read. I like to cook. I like to sew. I like to watch movies. I can't fit all of those things into every day, especially with juggling a day job, a newspaper column, and other writing assignments and speaking engagements.

So what would I do if on top of being busy, I didn't like to exercise? That is a poser. I think that a lot of people who don't like exercise just haven't found the right activity. For every person who adores yoga or running or salsa dancing, there are a hundred others who consider that activity a form of torture. For most people, physical activity can be fun, so in the interest of health and all the other benefits movement brings, it's well worth it to test out different activities to find the ones that fit.

The core of my activity routine is walking and weight lifting. I have a stationary bike for when the weather is sucky. I enjoy yoga for its mental and physical aspects (and because it feels good!), but it's an accessory exercise for me. When the weather is fine, I like to work some hikes into my schedule because of the added benefits of exercising in nature.

Why do I make the time to exercise? Or, maybe the better question is how? I've committed to exercising regularly, and being strong and flexible with good endurance aligns with many of my core values, including being independent. I also like to sightsee on foot when I travel, so I often view long walks at home as "training for travel." Lifting weights also makes it easier to haul my luggage out of metro stations that don't have escaltors! Exercise is something I just do, and while it certainly doesn't define me, it's become one part of who I am.

Why exercise needs a PR makeover

THE TWO TIMES OF THE YEAR most likely to nudge non-exercisers to start exercising is the new year, with its new round of resolutions, and spring, with its reminder that we'll soon be wearing fewer layers of clothing when we're out in public. Unfortunately, the renewed interest in moving more is typically tied to weight rather than wellness. I blame a societal publicity campaign fueled by "fat burning" magazine articles, gym marketing, and public health messages.

It is time to decouple exercise from weight loss. While there is abundant evidence for the benefits of nutritious food for health and well-being, the evidence is even stronger for the regular physical activity. That's true for all people, of all ages, of all weights. But the unfortunate fact remains that many people who aim to improve their eating and exercise habits view it as a means to an end: a lower number on the scale and a smaller size on the clothing rack. Here are three comments about exercise I hear repeatedly, and why they work against us:

"I did a six-week boot camp and didn't lose any weight, so I stopped going." The means to an end mindset can lead to abandonment of new food- and fitness-related health habits if they don't produce weight loss. Weight is a poor long-term motivator, in part because there's no guarantee you'll reach your goal. Health is a better goal, and cultivating a deeper value of self-care. It's easy to think exercise isn't "doing anything" because it's not leading to weight loss, but the truth it is doing a lot—just deep inside, where you can't see it.

"If my exercise doesn't make me feel like I'm going to die/throw up/pass out, it's not worth doing." This is the retooled version of "feel the burn" or "no pain, no gain." Some people love spin class, while for others it's a special form of hell. Yet I know people who fall in the second camp who feel like they "should" do spin class because it burn more calories. Ditto for joyful walkers who feel they "should" run, even though they hate it. Instead of focusing on burning calories, choose types of activity that make you feel good and bring you joy. That will help keep you motivated.

"My weight is fine, so I don't need to exercise." Exercise has been called the most efficient way to maintain health, and has countless benefits for mind and body—at all body weights. In our weight-focused culture, weight has become shorthand for health, but research shows that endurance, muscle strength, flexibility and balance are important for reducing the risk of chronic disease and staying physically independent as we age. Always-thin people who wait until they are diagnosed with type 2 diabetes to form a physical activity habit will find themselves behind the eight ball.

Even better, exercise has been shown to expand our brain volume and strengthen our neural networks—including those that are associated with habit formation. This may be why many people find it easier to eat healthfully when they're exercising regularly. The brain changes that happen when we form one healthy habit may "transfer" to another habit. Dismissing exercise because it doesn't change your body size means you'll miss out not only on its inherent health benefits, but you'll miss the benefits of its positive spillover into other areas of your life. So how will you move today?

The 3-legged stool of fitness

WHAT DO YOU THINK of when you think of exercise or physical activity? Running or walking? Gym workouts? Yoga? Those are all great examples (but not the only examples). More importantly, together they paint a picture of what a well-balanced exercise routine looks like: endurance, and flexibility. I call this the Three-Legged Stool of Fitness. Leave one out, and your stool will topple!

- **Endurance.** Also known as cardiovascular or aerobic exercise, endurance exercise builds endurance by working your heart and lungs. Classic examples include running/jogging, brisk walking, aerobics or Zumba classes, swimming, biking, cross-country skiing and elliptical machines. For this type of exercise to "count," you need to be working at a pace that makes it a little difficult, but not impossible, to carry on a conversation.
- **Strength.** As I mentioned, once you pass age 30, you start to lose lean muscle mass unless you make a point of preserving it. While eating adequate protein at each meal is important for keeping, or building, muscle, strength training is hands down the best way to stay strong. While lifting weights (with free weights or machines) is the classic ex-

ample of strength training, providing resistance with body weight exercises like pushups, lunges, planks and squats or with stretchy bands or tubes can also build strength. Even if you prefer to use weights, bands and tubes are a good way to stay strong while traveling. When you're 20, 30, 40, 50 and maybe even 60, you don't think about becoming frail. You don't think about losing your muscle mass. But you should think about it, because it's at those ages that you can take steps to protect your muscle. How are your muscles? Are you actively working to keep them? If not, start now.

- **Flexibility.** Although some people are naturally more flexible than others, there is value to actively maintaining (or slightly improving upon) what nature gave you. Gently stretching your muscles, tendons, ligaments and other connective tissue feels good, and is also good for you. While I haven't seen any research specifically on this topic, I suspect that incorporating flexibility exercises into your routine may be even more important if you find yourself sitting at a desk much of the day, as many modern workers do. Yoga is a classic, and more formalized, way to improve flexibility, but garden-variety stretches will do, too. In case you haven't heard, it's a myth that you need to stretch before doing other exercise.

Of course, many types of physical activity incorporate elements of more than one of these categories. Walking or running build endurance and cardiovascular fitness while strengthening your leg muscles (although not all leg muscles are worked evenly, fyi). Yoga can help build strength as you move your body through different poses (but how much strength will depend on how active or vigorous your form of yoga is). Strength or resistance training may aid flexibility if you are moving your joints and muscles through a full range of motion.

Are you balanced?

Arguably, you could add a fourth leg to the Three-Legged Stool of Fitness: Balance. Each of us has our own innate sense of balance, but no matter where we start from, we can improve. Improving and maintaining balance becomes very important with age, as poor balance can make daily activity more difficult and increase the risk of falls and fractures. But people of all ages can benefit from improving their balance. As with many things, it's never too late to start boosting your balance, but earlier is better than later! I encourage making it a point to incorporate balance-improving moves in almost every activity you do:

- **Walking.** This may not seem like it has anything to do with balance, but have you ever watched someone who is extremely sedentary (due to advanced age or serious illness) try to walk? They look like they are in danger of falling over at any second. Balance is a multifaceted thing that involves many parts of you (muscles, nerves, inner ear, etc.) working together to keep you properly oriented in space. The simple act of going for regular walks helps support that.
- **Free weights.** When you opt for free weights (or body weight) over machines for your strength training, you gain more than just muscle tone and strength, you gain balance. There are no machine parts holding things in a certain place…it's all up to you. I like to up the ante by incorporating moves that challenge my balance further: one-legged deadlifts and squats, lunges and stability ball exercises.
- **Yoga.** This is a great way to progressively improve your balance. Simpler moves like the warrior poses require some balance, but harder moves like tree pose, half-moon pose and standing splits will make all but the balance savants wobble like a weeble at first. When you finally can hold these poses for a reasonable length of time, it's pretty exhilarating!
- **Dance.** Many forms of dance require balance, especially when you get beyond practicing basic moves and start practicing choreography. Some styles of dance have you up on your toes a lot, which is of course challenging at first if your balance isn't so hot.
- **Martial arts.** I haven't studied martial arts (other than dabbling in one Tai Chi class many, many years ago), but I'm guessing that those would do quite a bit for balance, too.

Formal exercise aside, there is something to be said for incorporating little bouts of balance into your day-to-day life. Practice standing on one foot while waiting in line, brushing your teeth, talking on the phone. It may seem silly, but do it enough, and the benefits will accrue.

The mental benefits of movement

Physical activity is good for your body, sure, but don't underestimate what it can do for your mental outlook. Exercise, especially when done regularly, is a powerful way to help keep stress levels at a management level. I've also noticed that I do some of my best thinking while moving (the rest of my great thinking happens in the shower, naturally).

I don't advise trying to think too much while lifting weights (research has shown that you actually have a more effective workout if you focus on the movements you are doing), but walks are a fantastic vehicle for clearing your head or brainstorming ideas. I can't even tell you how many times I've had a great insight while walking. An idea for a blog post. The perfect approach for an article I'm writing. What to make for dinner. How to reverse climate change and achieve world peace. You get the idea. Is it any wonder that many companies that foster a culture of health also endorse holding "walking meetings"?

When it comes to mind-body benefits of physical activity, you may automatically think of yoga. Even though I yoga is fantastic for this purpose, it's important to remember that almost any form of exercise can contribute mental benefits. Our bodies are meant to move, and if we don't move them, our bodies are not the only thing that will suffer!

Finding time to move

DO YOU OBSESS ABOUT what time is the "best time" to exercise? True, you can get bogged down in details about whether you burn slightly more calories or your strength and endurance is just a little bit greater at a certain time of day. But the greater truth is this: The best time to exercise is the time you actually do it!

I need to exercise early in the day, or there is an extreme danger that I won't exercise at all. On weekdays, that means weightlifting or yoga before work, and a walk at lunch. Ironically, I find it harder to exercise on the weekend, when my days are less structured and it's easy to get caught up in other absorbing projects (cleaning, gardening, cooking, studying) until suddenly it's evening and my exercise window closes with a slam.

I know that on weekends I need to just out of bed and go for a walk, yet I seldom do this in the winter when mornings are dark and cold. Often, I do end up going for a walk in the afternoon…but not always. It's a classic case of knowing what to do, but not doing it. We can so easily fool ourselves that things will somehow fall into place, even though experience tells us otherwise. When it comes to healthy living, and other areas of life, for that matter, we would be much better off if we could find a way to consistently act in ways that honor what we know to be true about our best selves.

When I do fit a walk, weight lifting or yoga into my morning, it's always a great start to my day. Once I'm done, it feels fantastic to have crossed a major to-do off my list. I've put my muscles through their paces and feel like I really "earned" my morning cup of coffee. Finally, and perhaps most importantly, I enjoy the satisfaction that comes from turning intention into action.

I find that as the day goes on, there is a greater risk that one of my other "likes" will kick exercise off the daily schedule. That's why I tend to exercise in the mornings, when the day is fresh. (I've often noticed that early morning outdoor exercisers are a cheerful lot…it's a bit like being in an exclusive club, or knowing the secret handshake).

I love the feeling of exercise, but that doesn't mean that making time for exercise always comes easy. I might be pressed for time, or tired, or distracted, or whatever. But 99 times out of 100, if I can make myself put on my workout clothes, lace up my shoes, and start exercising, my head (and the rest of me) gets in the game. I know that's not only true for me… so I bet it's true for you, too.

Beyond "formal" exercise

Think hitting the gym on the way home makes up for the hours you just spent sitting at a desk and the evening you will spend sitting on the couch watching the tube? Think again! For the last several years, I've been reading with interest the growing body of research showing that sitting, sitting and more sitting is not very good for us.

The Mayo Clinic's James Levine, who does research about non-exercise activity thermogenesis (NEAT), otherwise known as the calories you burn through movement other than intentional exercise (walking to lunch, cleaning the house, pacing while talking on the phone) says that being sedentary for hours a day (a common occurrence for anyone who has a desk job) can work against health whether or not you go to the gym or get formal exercise that day. I've said it before, and I'll say it again: Our bodies are meant to move. And not just in one big dose every day or every other day. Another inactivity researcher, Marc Hamilton, says it clearly:

"Exercise is not a perfect antidote for sitting."

Even if you have to work at a desk all day, try to move for a few minutes ever hour or hour-and-a-half. This also has mental benefits, as research shows that our mental sharpness dips if we focus on one task for too long.

I do most of my exercise before work, but I also go for a short walk at lunch. I take the train home from work, so I get about 1.5 miles of walking before I make dinner and settle into an evening of reading or writing.

At work, I get up from my desk between patients, but if I do find myself potentially sitting for a stretch, I make it a point to get up roughly once an hour. To be perfectly honest, my habit of drinking a lot of water makes this easy, both from the input and output sides of the equation, if you catch my drift, and I think that you do.

Chapter summary

Who doesn't want to be strong and able to do the things they want to do? The good news is that with exercise and adequate protein, you have a lot of power in staying fit for (your) life.

Here are the main takeaways from Chapter 6:

- You get maximum benefit from protein when you spread it throughout your day.
- The power of plant proteins to improve your muscles, your nutrition and your health is quite mighty.
- It's a myth that we get too much protein, and that protein is hard on our kidneys and leaches calcium from our bones.
- To be consistently active, you need to find ways to move that bring you joy, and to figure out what motivates you.
- As with nutrition, variety is important in exercise. Incorporate activities for endurance, strength and flexibility.
- Knowing yourself, and redefining what exercise means, are two ways to make sure exercise happens.

Coming up in Chapter 7, Fuel and Fiber:

- Carbohydrates and your body
- Whole grain goodness
- Celiac disease and gluten sensitivity
- Preparing whole grains
- Natural vs. Added sugar
- Kicking the SSB habit

Fuel and Fiber

WHERE ONCE FAT was demonized, now carbs are Public Enemy Number One with many people. The truth is that carbs are not the devil! Carbs are an important source of energy and, yes, pleasure! But as with food in general, quality is key. Not all carbs are created equal. Some carbohydrate-rich foods are nutritious and beneficial to health, while others are not so much—and deserve a much smaller role in our overall way of eating.

In this chapter, i'll talk about:

- **Carbohydrates and your body.** In other word, what have carbs done for us lately.
- Not convinced? I'll do some grain myth-busting and get you excited about **whole grain goodness.**
- While most people don't need to avoid gluten (it's true), those with **celiac disease and gluten sensitivity** do need to avoid or limit gluten-containing grains.
- OK, so you're on board with whole grains…now what? I won't leave you hanging! I'll give you the basics about **preparing whole grains.**
- There's been a lot of harsh talk about sugar lately, and most of it is deserved. Still, I see a lot of confusion about **natural vs. added sugar,** which I will happily clear up for you.
- Why SSBs are perhaps the worst way to ingest sugar, plus tips for kicking the SSB habit.

Carbohydrates and your body

WHAT IS A CARBOHYDRATE? In simplest terms, carbohydrates are made up of carbon, oxygen and hydrogen atoms. Water (which is hydrating) is made of oxygen and hydrogen, so when you add in the carbon you get "hydrate of carbon," which becomes the common term "carbohydrate."

Your body breaks down carbohydrates into glucose, which is a sci-ence-y name for sugar. This could give you pause, but it shouldn't. In ex-cess, sugar is not good for you, but the problems lie almost all with "add-ed sugar," those sugars added to everything from desserts to hamburger buns to jarred spaghetti sauce to sports drinks.

Your body uses glucose to create adenosine triphosphate (ATP), your body's "energy currency." (Think of glucose as a $100 bill that you need to break in order to be able to spend it in a store. ATP would be the smaller bills.) Every cell in your body uses glucose as its primary source energy, and your brain in particular is a glucose hog. So it's not about avoiding sugar—it's about making sure our sugar comes in its natural packaging in the form of fruit, vegetables, grains and beans. Those are the major carbohydrate-containing foods.

In one sense, all carbohydrates are created equal, because all digestible carbohydrates are broken down into glucose. However, although there are some meaningful differences various carbohydrates based on how the basic building blocks are assembled.

Simple carbohydrates

Monosaccharides, or simple sugars, are the smallest type of carbohydrate. The most common monosaccharide is glucose, followed by fructose and galactose. We don't find many monosaccharides in food. What we do find are disaccharides, which are two monosaccharides joined together. Su-crose (glucose + fructose), also known as table sugar, is the most common disaccharide. Lactose (galactose + glucose), the natural sugar found in milk, is also common.

Complex carbohydrates

Oligosaccharides are short chains of three to nine monosaccharides. Polysaccharides are long chains of 10 or more monosaccharides. Some polysaccharides include hundreds or thousands of monosaccharides. From a nutrition point of view, the other important polysaccharides are starch, the storage carbohydrate of plants, and cellulose, a thick, strong fi-ber that gives fruits and vegetables their structure. All whole plant foods, including fruits, vegetables, grains, beans, nuts and seeds contain cellulose, which is a form of dietary fiber. Both starch and cellulose are entirely made of glucose.

Carbohydrates and digestion

In your small intestine (which is attached to your stomach on one end and your large intestine on the other), digestive enzymes break down dietary starches and disaccharides into monosaccharides, which are then absorbed by cells in your intestinal wall. Generally, the shorter the chain the quicker the digestion, but this depends partly on what other foods you eat in the same meal. Bacteria in your large intestine digest oligosaccharides. Cellulose passes through your body undigested, because humans don't have the right enzymes to break them down. (Some people with irritable bowel syndrome have trouble digesting oligosaccharides and other types of carbohydrates, which can cause gas and bloating.)

Whole grain goodness

THERE'S A LOT OF FEAR-MONGERING about carbohydrates in general, and grains in particular—even whole grains. Allow me to do a little bit of myth-busting.

First, carbohydrates are not evil. They aren't even bad. Carbs started to get a bad rap in the unfortunate aftermath of the low-fat era, when people started cutting back on fat and adding carbohydrates—refined carbohydrates in particular (aka sugar, white flour and products made from them). Depending on your age, you may have vivid memories of store shelves filled with green boxes of Snackwells cookies. Many people freely devoured entire boxes, thinking it was OK because they were fat-free (or nearly so).

The scientific and medical community never intended for people to replace fat with refined carbohydrates. They intended people to replace saturated fat with healthier sources of fat (like nuts, avocados, fatty fish, olive oil) and nutritious carbohydrates (whole grains, starchy and non-starchy vegetables, fruit). Unfortunately, this wasn't made clear, and food manufacturers decided to simplify the message to serve their marketing purposes, making all fat the devil, all carbs the angel, and doing a number on our health over the ensuing decades.

Eating more whole grains (and fewer refined grains), has been associated with a lower risk of major chronic diseases, such as heart disease and type 2 diabetes. A study published in January 2015 by researchers from the Harvard School of Public Health suggests that eating more whole grains is associated with a 15 percent lower chance of dying (that of course means dying earlier than you should due to disease and poor health...because each of us will die someday).

Grains in perspective

Certain books that I won't name here have blamed grains, including whole grains, for just about every health problem known to modern society. Some anti-grain advocates argue that humans did not evolve to eat grains. It's true that grain-based agriculture is a more recent part of our food history than, say, hunting for wooly mammoths, but it's not as recent as some people suggest. (If you want to watch a good TEDx talk on the topic, Google "Christina Warinner TED").

That said, grains may not agree with some people, but that doesn't mean that all people should avoid them. (Some people are allergic to nuts, that doesn't mean no one should eat nuts.) I personally know very healthy Paleo eaters (they eat starchy vegetables like sweet potatoes instead of grains) and very healthy vegetarians who eat whole grains as significant components of many meals (but limit refined grains).

The grain hierarchy

Full disclosure: I love bread. Good bread, specifically (sprouted whole-grain bread for toast or sandwiches, artisan sourdough to go with certain meals, fresh baguettes when in Paris). But while bread is definitely not the devil it's often made out to be, it's not the healthiest way to eat grains. No, that honor falls to intact whole grains.

Why intact whole grains? The simple truth is that once you grind whole grains into flour for bread, pasta or other products, it has become somewhat refined. Even though all parts of the grain (bran, germ, endosperm) are going to find their way into that product, the fact that they are ground up means that the carbohydrates will be absorbed more quickly into your bloodstream. Whole intact grains take longer to digest and absorb, which means they provide a steadier source of energy and are lower on the glycemic index (and therefore less inflammatory), especially when you eat them in a mixed meal or snack. Which brings me to...

No naked carbs!

Another relic of the low-fat era is the idea that snacking on pretzels or crackers is an ideal snack. Eating carbohydrate-rich foods (grains, starchy vegetables, fruit) by themselves allows their natural sugars to be digested and absorbed more rapidly. Yes, the fiber in whole fruit, and whole grains slows down this process, but for the steadiest energy release, and to prolong your post-eating feelings of satisfaction, it's best to eat carbohydrate foods with some protein and healthy fat. This can be as simple as:

- A few almonds with your apple (instead of just an apple)
- Some high-quality cheese with your crackers (instead of just crackers)
- A Greek yogurt with your granola bar (instead of just the bar)
- Adding Greek yogurt and protein powder to the fruit in your smoothie, and using almond milk instead of fruit juice

Celiac disease and gluten sensitivity

IS GOING GLUTEN-FREE a path to better health, or just another example of a fad diet? The answer depends on if you need to avoid gluten. Ironically, most people who avoid gluten don't need to, while most people who need to avoid gluten don't know they do.

Gluten is a type of protein found in wheat, rye and barley. Most of us can eat these grains without ill effects. However, a few of us can't, because we have a wheat allergy, celiac disease or non-celiac gluten sensitivity.

If you don't fall into one of these groups, there's no evidence that you should avoid gluten. The words "gluten free" on a food package don't translate to "healthy." They usually just mean "more expensive." Packaged gluten-free foods can be highly processed and full of sugar, fat and other less-healthful ingredients. Most are not enriched with vitamins and minerals.

It's estimated that fewer than 1 in 100 children have a wheat allergy, and about half will outgrow it before adulthood. If you have a wheat allergy, your body reacts badly to one (or more) of the many proteins found in wheat. This might include gluten. Symptoms appear within minutes or hours and can include skin rashes, intestinal discomfort, wheezing and anaphylaxis.

About 1 in 100 people have celiac disease and about 6 in 100 have gluten sensitivity. Celiac disease, an autoimmune disorder, is the more serious of the two, because eating gluten prompts the immune system to attack the lining of the small intestine. This causes damage that makes it harder for the body to absorb certain nutrients, including iron, calcium, vitamin D and folate. Down the road, this can lead to health problems like anemia and osteoporosis.

Celiac disease can only develop in genetically predisposed people, but carrying the genes isn't a guarantee you'll develop the disease. Potential symptoms include the classic intestinal problems, as well as weight changes, chronic fatigue and neurological problems. The only known treatment for celiac disease is total, lifelong avoidance of gluten. Even tiny amounts can cause intestinal damage and long-term problems. Gluten sensitivity has similar symptoms, but without the intestinal damage, so sufferers can usually be less strict.

Why is it that many people who need to avoid gluten don't know they need to? Often it's because their symptoms are mild or sort of vague. Even when symptoms are obvious, many other health conditions have similar symptoms, which can make diagnosis difficult. If you suspect you have celiac disease, get tested for the anti-gluten antibodies before you eliminate gluten. This increases the odds of an accurate test result. There is no test for gluten sensitivity, so diagnosis is based on ruling out other problems.

If you do need to avoid gluten, be sure to consider what you are eating as well as what you aren't eating. There are many healthful, naturally gluten-free foods, such as fruits and vegetables, beans, fish, nuts, eggs, yogurt, poultry, lean meat and gluten-free grains like quinoa and brown rice.

Preparing whole grains

IF YOU HAVE BEEN THINKING about experimenting with cooking whole grains—whether you've never cooked them at all, or want to branch out from brown rice and oatmeal—you may worry about getting the right grain-to-liquid proportion and the correct cooking time. Here, I'll try to make it easy for you!

Some grains take much longer to cook than others (you can download a cooking chart from the website). To avoid delaying dinner, plan accordingly. Many grains, like quinoa, bulgur, buckwheat and teff, cook in 30 minutes or less, so you can let them do their think while you prepare other parts of the meal.

For longer-cooking grains, try them out on the weekend when you have more lead time before dinner. Or, you can cook a batch ahead of time, keep it in the fridge (it will stay good for 3-4 days), then heat up some with a bit of broth or water when it's meal time. Leftover cooked whole grains are also great tossed into a salad with veggies, dressing, and a source of protein like cooked beans, canned tuna or leftover chicken.

Really, cooking grains is similar to cooking pasta, except that you put the grain and broth/water in a pot together before bringing it to a boil, whereas with pasta you bring the water to a boil first. If you ever forget how much liquid to add per cup of whole grain, you can always treat it like pasta—add lots of water and then simply drain the excess away when the grain is done to your preferred degree of tenderness.

Even when you know how much water and how much time, these measurements are simply guidelines. Many things affect how much time a grain takes to cook, including the variety of grain, how long it's been sitting in your pantry (or on the store shelf), and what type of pan or pot you're using. Always treat time as a guideline, not a rule:

If the time is up but the grain is not as tender as you might like, add a bit more water and keep cooking and testing until you're happy. If the grain seems done even though there's still time on your kitchen timer and the liquid isn't all absorbed, take the pot off the heat and drain the excess liquid.

Washing grains

I admit that I didn't pre-wash my grains (other than quinoa) until recently, when I was cooking with a professional chef and she gently scolded me and showed me how to wash rice. Washing grains takes a few extra minutes, but it's worth it. The fact is that grains can have hidden debris on them. The most important grains to wash are:

- Farro (which often has a dry, powdery coating)
- Rice (to remove excess starch)
- Quinoa (which may be covered with a powdery resin called saponin, which can taste bitter)

To wash your grains, put them in a large enough bowl to be able to cover them with lots of cold water. Repeatedly grab small handfuls of the grains (or seeds, in the case of quinoa) and rub them together. I like to do this, then carefully dump off most of the water, add new water, and repeat a few more times. When you're done, dump the grains into a fine mesh strainer and run more cold water over it as it drains freely.

Breakfast grains

There are few things as comforting and satisfying, especially on a chilly morning, as a bowl of hot oatmeal. But when it comes to cooking a pot of whole grains for breakfast, many people rarely make it past oats. That's a pity, because whole grains like quinoa, wild rice, wheat berries, bulgur and barley aren't just for dinner—they also deserve a place in your breakfast bowl.

Although exact nutrient profiles vary, whole grains are generally good-to-excellent sources of many B vitamins and several minerals. By including a variety of whole grains in your diet, you benefit from a more diverse array of nutrients than if you stick to just a few favorites. Most whole grains are also a good source of protein and a good-to-excellent source of fiber. Intact whole grains provide a slower, steadier release of energy (glucose) into your bloodstream than do grains that have been stripped of their outer bran, as is the case with white rice, or ground into flour for bread or pastries.

If you tend to feel better and stay satisfied longer when you eat a higher-protein breakfast, you can still include whole grains in your breakfast rotation. Quinoa, buckwheat, amaranth and hard wheat berries are good go-to grains, as they are highest in protein. To further boost protein, use milk for some of the cooking liquid, stir in an egg at the end of cooking, or finish with some nuts or a spoonful of nut butter.

To sweeten your breakfast grains, think beyond brown sugar and honey. Diced fresh fruit, mashed banana or dried fruit will provide natural sweetness as well as nutrients (be aware that some dried fruit has added sugar). Adding a dash of vanilla and a "baking" spice like cinnamon, nutmeg, ginger or cardamom can add aroma and the illusion of sweetness.

An easy way to start branching out at breakfast is with one of the multi-grain hot cereals from companies like Bob's Red Mill. Just follow the instructions on the package. Or, just pick a whole grain you like to cook for dinner, cook up a batch for breakfast, then dress it up like you would oatmeal. Cooking times for whole grains vary from 15 minutes to an hour. For most people, the longer cooking times are only realistic on weekend mornings—or in advance.

The great thing about cooked whole grains is that they reheat wonderfully with the addition of a little extra liquid. Leftover cooked grains from dinner can even be turned into breakfast the next morning, as long as you cook them in water and not a savory broth! This is a fantastic (and necessary) time-saver if you find you barely have time to make instant oatmeal in the morning. If you are caught in an instant oatmeal rut, switching to the less-processed thick cut or steel cut oats, or another whole grain, will probably feel more satisfying.

People with celiac disease or non-celiac gluten sensitivity need to avoid wheat, rye and barley…but what about oats? Although the oat itself does not contain gluten, oats are frequently contaminated with wheat during growing or processing. If your doctor says that pure, uncontaminated oats are OK for you, be sure to buy pre-packaged oats that are labeled gluten-free.

In a healthy diet, where does fruit fit?

THERE WAS A TIME when we didn't question whether fruit was good for us, when we more or less took the edict to "eat your fruits and veggies" to heart. Today, many people have developed a fear of fruit ("It has so much sugar!") while others arguably eat too much of it, forgetting about the veggies.

Fruit has a unique position in a healthy diet. In terms of nutrients, it's more like a vegetable. In terms of carbohydrate and calorie content it's more like a grain (or a starchy vegetable). Many dietitians and nutritionists groaned when Weight Watchers decided to make fruit a "free food."

From a nutrient standpoint, many fruits are rich in not just vitamins and minerals, but also phytonutrients, those natural plant-based compounds that may have a variety of health benefits, including cancer prevention and cardiovascular health. Pigment-rich berries and cherries, which are deliciously in season locally, are especially good sources of phytonutrients.

From a carbohydrate point of view, one slice of bread or 1/3 cup of cooked grain has roughly the same amount of carbohydrate as half of a large banana or 12 cherries. Fruit is certainly a more nutritious choice than refined grains, but it's no substitute for non-starchy vegetables like broccoli, cabbage, and dark leafy greens. I often hear, "I'm don't care for vegetables, but I eat lots of fruit!"

It's true that whole fruit contains a fair amount of sugar, but it's natural sugar, wrapped in a fiber-rich, water-rich, nutrient-rich package. That makes fruit is the healthiest sweet around, and we naturally like the taste of sweet because we were literally born with an affinity for it. However, if you struggle with sugar cravings, trading your candy and ice cream for lots of fruit will probably just keep feeding your raging sweet tooth.

So how much fruit should you eat? That depends. Generally speaking, people who have physically demanding jobs or participate in intense physical activity have higher carbohydrate needs, and fruit is a carbohydrate-rich food. People who sit at a desk most of the day and get minimal to moderate physical activity need less carbohydrate, and therefore less fruit.

As I already mentioned, something I say to my patients all the time is "No 'naked' carbs." In other words, don't eat a carbohydrate-rich food, such as fruit, by itself. A balanced meal or snack pairs carbohydrates with protein and healthy fat, slowing digestion enough to keep you satisfied and support healthy blood sugar levels. If you find that you are hungry soon after eating a "healthful" breakfast of oatmeal and fruit, it's likely because it's high in carbohydrates but low in protein—aka naked carbs. Here are a few examples of healthful, balanced ways to incorporate fruit into your day:

- Breakfast: Scrambled eggs or tofu with veggies and a side of fruit OR plain Greek yogurt with berries and nuts.
- Lunch: Tossed green salad with protein (chicken, fish, beef,

tofu or tempeh), healthy fat (nuts, seeds or avocado) an olive oil vinaigrette and a side of fruit.

- Dinner: One piece of fruit for dessert at the end of the meal.
- Snack: An apple with a small handful of nuts or a small piece of cheese, ½ large or one small banana with nut butter, ½ cup of plain Greek yogurt or cottage cheese with berries.

Kicking the SSB habit

OK, BY NOW YOU'VE probably heard that drinking sugar-sweetened beverages (SSBs) isn't the best thing for your waistline or your health. That includes soda, sports drinks and energy drinks as well as fruit juice. (Orange juice with pulp has a bit of fiber to partially redeem it, but juices like apple and grape are glorified sugar water).

The main problem with these beverages is that they deliver a lot of sugar and calories, quickly, without making us feel full. Diet soda is better than regular soda from a calorie point of view, but some research suggests that their intense sweetness may enhance appetite and contribute to an overall preference for sweet foods.

So what's a better beverage? Water. It quenches our thirst and hydrates our bodies without unnecessary extras. Trouble is, some people just do not like plain water. While "pure" water (H_2O) is flavorless, the water we encounter contains varying amounts of minerals and gases that give it flavor. That means tastiness is in the mouth of the drinker. As much as I love a cold glass of Seattle tap water, I don't always like the local water when I travel. For example, I can barely tolerate Las Vegas tap water. If you're not a water fan (or even if you are) try these tips for giving it a kick:

- **Go fruity.** Add a slice—or a squeeze— of lemon, lime or orange. (These are easy to pack in a baggie and tote to work, too.) Or, smash some berries and stir a spoonful in your glass.
- **Make iced tea.** Here's a tip I learned recently: In the morning before heading to work, drop a Lipton Cold Brew tea bag in a quart container of cold water. Once you get to work, remove the bag and you have a quart of iced tea to enjoy through the day.
- **Make personal sun tea.** Put two tea bags in a glass of water and set it on a sunny windowsill for 20 minutes. Pour over ice. This works with black, green or herbal teas.
- **Get exotic.** Float a slice of cucumber and a sprig of mint in your glass, or stir in a touch of pomegranate molasses (a

concentrated syrup of pomegranate juice and sugar). You can find it at grocers that sell Middle Eastern and Mediterranean foods. A teaspoon only has 40 calories—much better than a soda.

- **Be bubbly.** Mineral water, club soda or seltzer might appeal to you. Some people just don't like flat water and find that bubbles make it palatable.

What if you are in the habit of drinking several sodas a day, and switching to water—flavored or not—seems impossible? Try tapering off. Cut out one, then two, then three. If you feel that you have to go cold turkey, you may avoid making any changes at all.

So how much water should you be drinking? Research has kind of debunked the idea that there's a "right" amount, but eight 8-ounce glasses of fluid (not just water) per day is a rough minimum guideline. Try to drink when you're thirsty, and expect that you'll need to drink more during warm weather or when you're exercising.

Chapter summary

If you've been carrying around any lingering carb-phobia, I hope that this chapter has helped you to better understand the importance of carbs, generally, in a balanced, pleasurable diet, as well as which carbs contribute to health, and which, well, don't. Here are the main takeaways from Chapter 7:

Here are the main takeaways from Chapter 7:

- Your body needs carbohydrates.
- When it comes to carbs, quality counts if you want to feel your best and have steady energy, so embrace whole grains.
- Celiac disease and gluten sensitivity are serious, but if you don't have them, avoiding gluten is useless.
- The distinction between natural and added sugar is important, because they come in different nutritional packages.
- An occasional sugar-sweetened beverage (SSB) is no big deal, but it's worth it to kick the SSB habit, if you have one.

Coming up in Chapter 8, The Flavor Factor:

- Why you need fat
- What about coconut oil?
- Treat oils with TLC
- Nuts and seeds
- Spice it up for health

The Flavor Factor

FOOD MAY BE FUEL for our bodies, but let's face it, we want flavor, too! The good news is that nutritious food can absolutely be delicious and flavorful—I wouldn't have it any other way! While quality ingredients are a start for fuller flavor, smart use of spices, herbs and—yes!— fat are also important for mouthwatering meals.

In this chapter, I'll talk about:

- How to shed the vestiges of the unfortunate low fat era, and **why you need fat.**
- Clearing up confusion about what types of fat are good for us, and **putting saturated fat in (dietary) context.**
- Why the trans-fat ban is a double-edged sword.
- Why **coconut oil** is far from a cure for all that ails you, as some advocates would have you believe. Health halo alert!
- What happens when otherwise healthy fats "go bad," and why you should **treat oils with TLC.**
- The fact that **nuts and seeds** offer some of the healthiest, tastiest fats around, and why you should go nuts for nuts, without forgetting that seeds also offer good nutrition in a tiny package.
- Claiming maximum nutrition and flavor by **spicing it up for health.** I'll take you on a tour of the global spice pantry to give you a head start on elevating the ordinary.

Why you need fat

HOW DO YOU FEEL ABOUT FAT? Do you fear it? Do you treat it as an indulgence to be limited? With all the ups and downs in fat's status ("It's bad!" "It's good!" "No, wait, it's bad!") I would not be surprised at all if you had a little bit of dietary fat whiplash.

One cause for confusion is the oversimplification of how fat is discussed in the media. Fat is really a very complex thing. Not only do you have saturated and unsaturated (polyunsaturated and monounsaturated) fats, which can have different effects on health, but not all fats in one category (sat, mono, poly) are the same. To try to explain it simply, it's because one fat molecule (a triglyceride) is made up of three fatty acids attached to a glycerol "backbone" (three = "tri" and glycerol = "glyceride"). While all saturated fatty acids are straight, they come in different lengths. Different saturated fatty acids have different lengths (not to get too science-y, but fatty acids are chains of carbon atoms with hydrogen atoms attached) and that means have different effects on our blood cholesterol and triglyceride levels. While all unsaturated fatty acids have at least one bend in them, they also come in different lengths and the bends can be in different places. You may be going, "Huh?" but trust me, this makes a difference.

This is why it's too simple to say that "too much fat is bad" or "all saturated fats are bad and all unsaturated fats are good." The bottom line is that we all need fat in our diets but some fats are better for us than others. Most experts now agree that it's not about how much fat we eat, but what kind of fat we eat plus what we're eating besides fat!

Putting saturated fat in (dietary) context

Does saturated fat contribute to heart disease? This question is not easily answered. When you think of saturated fat, what's the first food that comes to mind? Odds are, it's beef or bacon. Would it surprise you to know that the top sources of saturated fat in the American diet are cheese, pizza, grain-based desserts and dairy-based desserts?

Foods high in both fat and sugar appeal to our taste buds and make up many of our food choices. This makes it even more difficult to tease out what role, if any, saturated fat may play in disease. We do know that cutting back on saturated fat isn't inherently healthy—it depends on what you replace it with.

Replacing saturated fat with polyunsaturated and monounsaturated fats is heart-healthy. Mediterranean-style diets are a prime example, as they are low in saturated fat, but not low in total fat, thanks to olive oil, nuts and fatty fish. (Interestingly, most unprocessed meats contain almost as much monounsaturated fats as they do saturated fats.)

On the other hand, a low-fat, high-carbohydrate diet may not be heart healthy, especially if it includes a lot of refined carbohydrates like sugar and white flour. We know that sugars, fructose in particular, are easily oxidized (oxidation is sort of like rust), which isn't good for us. We saw this scenario play out in the decades where low-fat diets were king, and consumption of big plates of pasta and whole boxes of SnackWells cookies abounded.

One thing I'm happy about is that nutrition research is starting to move away from looking at specific nutrients (including macronutrients like fat) and looking at the whole foods that those nutrients come packaged in. This means that whether saturated fat has positive, negative or neutral health effects may depend on what food it comes in. For example, research suggests that eating moderate amounts of full-fat dairy in the form of plain yogurt and quality cheese (very European!) has benefits for health. The fact that yogurt and cheese are both fermented foods may be one explanation.

While our food choices do matter if we want to prevent heart disease, decades of morphing and evolving science have helped us understand that a "whole diet" approach—paying attention to what you do eat as well as what you don't—is more effective. To that end:

- **Go for quality over quantity.** There is a difference between getting your saturated fat from grass-fed beef or pastured pork from healthy animals than it is to get it in the form of an industrial beef patty, hotdog or pepperoni.
- **Aim for balance.** Serve that tasty grass-fed beef with a large tossed salad (with olive oil vinaigrette) or a pile of roasted vegetables…or both!
- **Embrace variety.** Mix up your protein choices to include more than just red meat: chicken, fish, beans and lentils.
- **Cook low and slow.** Meat contains small amounts of poly-unsaturated fats and carbohydrates, and these substances may be easily oxidized when cooked at high heats. Slow, lower heat cooking methods like stewing, braising or oven roasting may be healthier than grilling, broiling or frying.

The trans fat ban: a double-edged sword?

The Food and Drug Administration (FDA) ruled in June 2015 to ban trans fats, otherwise known as partially hydrogenated oils, from our food supply. That's a good thing, because trans fats, once hailed as a healthier alternative to saturated fats, have more recently been called "metabolic poison" by many health and nutrition experts, citing their role in heart disease and type 2 diabetes risk.

A trans fat is a liquid vegetable oil (unsaturated fat) that has been bombarded with extra hydrogen atoms (hydrogenation) to make it semi-solid at room temperature, closer to a solid saturated fat like butter or animal fat.

Because saturated fats were linked to heart disease and unsaturated fats were known to be heart-healthy, trans fats were supposed to offer the best of both worlds: Heart-healthy unsaturated fats with the culinary properties of saturated fats. As anyone who likes to bake knows, some recipes require a solid fat.

As it turns out, once unsaturated fats are hydrogenated, they are no longer heart-healthy. In fact, trans fats are even worse for heart health than saturated fats were ever believed to be. Clinical trials have shown that while saturated fats can raise "bad" LDL cholesterol, trans fats both raise LDL and lower "good" HDL cholesterol.

Although some experts expressed concern about trans fats early on, it took decades before mounting scientific evidence revealed trans fats' true nature. In the meantime, trans fats had seeped into all areas of food preparation. Restaurants were frying in partially hydrogenated oils instead of beef fat. Home cooks got the message that margarine was heart-healthy and that butter was not. It became rare to find a cracker, cookie, coffee creamer, frosting or mass-produced bakery item that didn't contain partially hydrogenated oil.

While the trans fat ban is a good thing, there is some concern about what might take the place of partially hydrogenated oils in processed foods. Could the ban be a double-edged sword?

For commercial frying, partially hydrogenated oils are simply being replaced by vegetable oils that are stable at high heat. But to replace solid fats, such as those used for baking and spreads, the trend so far is to produce trans fat-free shortenings using either palm oil or interesterified vegetable oil.

Palm oil is a tropical oil that comes from the fruit portion of the palm fruit. Most health and nutrition experts agree that this saturated fat is a lesser evil than trans fats, but it's unclear what effect palm oil may have on blood cholesterol and heart disease—good, bad or neutral. Interesterified oils have been used since the 1930s, including as a replacement for cocoa butter in cheap chocolate, but interest in them increased as the trans fat backlash began. The concern is that these chemically altered oils may have the same negative effects on our cholesterol and blood sugar levels as trans fats.

What can you do now until we know more about these fats? First, don't assume that the words "trans fat free" means that a food is nutritious. Second, if you eat more whole foods and fewer processed foods, you'll naturally be eating less of whatever type of fat is used in place of trans fats. This means you will be less affected if years from now it turns out that these trans fat alternatives aren't any better for us.

What about coconut oil?

COCONUT OIL ISN'T ANYTHING NEW, but it has become increasingly trendy over the last several years. While proponents of this tropical oil tout its real and imagined health benefits, detractors caution that coconut oil is a saturated fat, and saturated fat has been linked to heart disease. Who's right, and who's wrong? As is often the case, the truth is somewhere in the middle.

The original bad press about coconut oil started decades ago, based on studies that used partially hydrogenated coconut oil. Hydrogenated oils contain trans fats, which (as you just read) are very bad for our health. You won't find trans fats in the virgin coconut oil on store shelves, but you will find almost 90 percent saturated fat. That's the source of the current bad press.

The debate rages on about what saturated fat means for our health, exactly. As I mentioned, the answer may depend largely on what we eat instead of saturated fat. If you fill the calorie gap with hydrogenated oils or refined carbohydrates (sugar and white flour), that's not good. If you swap saturated fat for olive oil, which is rich in healthful monounsaturated fats, that is good.

Plus, remember that not all saturated fats are built from the same types of fatty acids.

There are a lot of health claims about coconut oil, mostly based on the fact that it contains what are called medium-chain fatty acids (MCTs). These supposedly are more beneficial from the long-chain saturated fatty acids that you find in fats from animal foods, but those claims are not supported by science, for two reasons:

1. The claims draw on research done on isolated MCTs, but coconut oil is mostly made of lauric acid, the longest of the medium-chain fatty acids. In the body, it actually behaves more like a long-chain saturated fatty acid.
2. Much research on coconut oil is specifically based on decades-old studies of indigenous populations studies who didn't use coconut oil in large amounts—they were using co-

conut flesh or squeezed coconut cream as part of their traditional diet, which of course was low in processed foods.

Removing nutrition and health from the equation for a moment, what are the culinary merits of coconut oil? Coconut oil is solid at room temperature, so it can be used in place of other solid fats like butter or shortening. This makes it great addition to the kitchen for vegan bakers and others who don't eat dairy products. While you can buy unscented coconut oil, many brands have a wonderful aroma and flavor that particularly lends itself to baking and Thai cuisine.

Coconut oil is often touted as having a high smoke point. The truth is that at 350°F, it's not super high, so don't use it for high-heat cooking. When you heat oils past their smoke point, they start to degrade, which isn't good for you

Here's the bottom line: If you enjoy coconut oil and find it a useful addition to your kitchen, use it in place of other saturated fats, not in addition to them.

5 myths—and facts—about olive oil

OLIVE OIL—ESPECIALLY EXTRA-VIRGIN OLIVE OIL (EVOO)—has earned a lot of respect for its integral role in the Mediterranean diet and for its health-promoting phytonutrients, antioxidants and monounsaturated fats. Olive oil is also unique among oils because it's essentially fruit juice—the olive "fruit" is mechanically crushed to extract the "juice." This is quite different from the process used to extract oil from seeds like canola, sunflower and safflower, which usually involves chemical solvents. Despite its healthfulness, there are several myths that cast a bit of a cloud over olive oil. Allow me to bust a few of them:

One: Most olive oil is adulterated. This myth stems from reports published by the University of California Davis several years ago suggesting that more than two-thirds of EVOO sold in California did not meet the quality criteria to justify the name. EVOO has to have some fruitiness and be free of defects like fustiness (when the olives start to ferment before pressing), mustiness (when olives start to mold before pressing) or rancidity (which means the oil started to oxidize before or during processing).

UC Davis found that two-thirds of the oils labeled EVOO did not meet these standards. Unfortunately, this has been widely misinterpreted to mean that the "failed" oils were adulterated with either inferior olive oil or with other oils like canola. So how did this disconnect happen? I had a chance to ask Dan Flynn, executive director of the UC Davis Olive Center. "It partly got misinterpreted because it's easier in the media to report that something's fake," he said. "It also plays into the bigger story about inauthenticity in food." He also suspects that many people who wrote about the report didn't actually read it.

The North American Olive Oil Association (NAOOA) guards against adulteration through random testing. While there are rare instances of adulteration, the NAOOA's testing of hundreds of bottles each year confirms that it's actually a very rare occurrence today.

Two: It's not healthy to cook with EVOO. Think that olive oil isn't safe to use above moderate heats? Think again. EVOO loses some of its unique flavor during cooking, but it doesn't become unhealthy. While it's true that EVOO has a lower "smoke point" (the point when an oil starts to smoke and break down) than refined oils like canola oil, vegetable oils and light olive oil, it's high enough to be a healthful choice for almost all types of cooking we do at home. Mediterranean countries, especially Greece, cook everything in extra-virgin olive oil.

The truth is that smoke point depends partly on the quality, age and condition of the oil. Good-quality EVOO is safe in a range of 350-410 degrees F, in part because it is rich in antioxidants, which protect the oil from becoming damaged when heated. Poor quality oil, or oil that has gone rancid, will have a lower smoke point.

Three: You can tell a quality olive oil by looking at it. Quality olive oil isn't a generic product. According to the NAOOA, variance based on factors like olive variety, growing conditions and country of origin creates variability in oil color—from pale yellow to dark green—and how fast the oil will cloud or solidify in the refrigerator. While an oil's color is worth admiring, but it says nothing about the quality of the oil, or the flavor. Many people think, that greener oils have a peppery flavor, while golden oils are more "buttery." Not necessarily true.

Four: It matters where olive oil comes from. Less than 4 percent of the olive oil consumed in this country is actually produced here—with most of the rest coming from Mediterranean countries. California produces about 99 percent of domestic olive oil. It's a mistake to assume that an olive oil is good just because it comes from, say, Italy or Greece or California. "The origin in terms of the state or country is not that important from the standpoint of quality," Flynn said. "Quality comes down to the producer level. Just because olive oil has been made somewhere for a long time doesn't mean that everything that comes out of that place is going to be great."

Five: Olive oil gets better with age. Flynn says that a quality oil should last two years from when it was bottled, provided that it is stored in a capped bottle away from light and heat, and that a harvest date on the bottle is often a good indicator of quality. "The fact that a producer cares that a consumer knows when the oil was harvested tends to indicate that the producer is 'above the bar,'" he said. Shoppers can also look for quality seals from the NAOOA, USDA, California Olive Oil Council or the Extra Virgin Alliance.

Treat oils with TLC

ANY DISCUSSION OF DIETARY FAT and health should go beyond how much fat to eat, and what types. It should also consider best practices for purchasing, storing and using fats and oils.

The most healthful high-fat foods include fish, nuts, seeds, olives and avocados. Not surprisingly, some of the healthiest oils come from these foods. I recommend buying the best quality you can afford of any food, whether it be carrots or cookies, but quality is especially important with fats and the foods that contain them.

First, choose organic, unrefined, cold-pressed oils whenever you can. Many pesticides are fat soluble, which means they accumulate in fat. In addition, many mass-produced vegetable oils are subjected to chemicals and high heat during processing.

It can help to remember high-quality oils are more than just fat. They also contain many of the healthful compounds that were found in the fruit, nut or seed they came from. How you store and use these oils is important, because light, air, heat and time can degrade them, destroying their nutrients and turning them rancid, at which point you should throw them away. Store oils in a cool, dry place away from direct light, and sniff before using to check for unpleasant or "off" odors.

Finally, not all oils and fats respond the same way to heat. Some don't like heat at all, others can handle high heat. When oil goes rancid, either because of overheating or poor storage conditions, healthful antioxidants in the oil also degrade. This can turn them into unhealthful—even dangerous—free radicals. (It's even worse if you reheat and reuse vegetable oils.) Here are my top picks for which oils to use at various temperatures:

- **High heat.** Not many healthful oils will stand up to these temperatures. As mentioned, a quality extra-virgin olive oil will have enough antioxidants to protect the oil from the heat. Unrefined "virgin" avocado oil is another sturdy oil with lots of good fats. A refined high-oleic sunflower oil isn't my top pick generally, but it not the worst choice and it can take the heat.
- **Medium-high heat.** EVOO is still a go-to here, as is avo-

112

cado oil. Peanut oil is another good choice. Feel free to use sesame or virgin, unrefined coconut oil for dishes where their unique flavors would be complimentary.

- **Low or medium heat (including baking).** Extra-virgin olive oil is still a top pick here (I use it in baking all the time, and my muffins never taste like olives). Because coconut oil is solid at room temperature, it can work well for baked goods that need a solid fat. Butter fits here too, where the flavor or texture are needed.
- **No heat.** Flaxseed oil is rich in a number of healthful compounds, including heart-healthy omega-3s. This makes it fragile, so store it in the fridge and never heat it. Use it to dress salads or already-cooked vegetables. Treat healthful hemp seed oil and unrefined hazelnut or walnut oils similarly.

Nuts and seeds

MANY PEOPLE FALL INTO one of two camps about nuts and seeds. Either they are hesitant to fully include them in their meals and snacks because they are high in calories and fat, or they are fully on board with the facts that fat is not the enemy AND that nuts and seeds provide healthy fats, only to end up going overboard with them.

Yes, overdoing the nuts and seeds may provide you with more calories than your body needs, but, no, avoiding them altogether is not necessary! In fact, research shows that people who eat nuts tend to have healthier body weights and be less likely to gain weight (there's not as much research about seeds and body weight, but we can probably make the same connection). This may be because nuts are satiating and some of the calories in nuts are inefficiently absorbed.

While exact nutrient compositions vary, nuts and seeds are rich sources of heart-healthy fats, fiber, plant protein, essential vitamins and minerals, and other bioactive compounds, including an array of phytonutrients that appear to have antioxidant and anti-inflammatory benefits.

Consider using nuts and seeds as a substitute for other protein-containing foods, instead of just an addition to your diet. Sprinkle on salads or sautéed veggies. Add to your morning oatmeal or cold cereal. Mix some into yogurt. Add to baked goods or homemade granola. Because of their high fat content, seeds benefit from being stored in an airtight container in a cool, dark place, ideally in the refrigerator, or even the freezer.

Go Nuts for Nuts

A wealth of research suggests that eating tree nuts reduces the risk of several chronic diseases, including cardiovascular disease, type 2 diabetes and some forms of cancer. There may be benefits for brain health, as well. Adding support to these findings is research suggesting that including tree nuts in your diet reduces the risk of health conditions such as high blood pressure, high cholesterol, insulin resistance, abdominal obesity and inflammation.

Various components of nuts, such as heart-healthy fats (monounsaturated, polyunsaturated and omega-3 fatty acids), high-quality protein, fiber, vitamins (including folate, niacin and vitamin E), minerals (including potassium, calcium and magnesium) and phytonutrients (carotenoids, flavonoids, polyphenols and phytosterols) may work together to promote health.

Research results suggest that a Mediterranean diet that includes a serving of nuts per day protects against heart attack, stroke or death from other cardiovascular causes in people at high risk for these serious health problems due to type 2 diabetes or metabolic syndrome. Data also suggests that eating more than three servings of nuts per week reduces risk of premature death from all causes, especially when also following a Mediterranean diet. People who frequently eat both nuts and walnuts were less likely to die from cancer.

The evidence is substantial enough that dietary guidelines in the United States, Canada and other countries recommend including nuts as part of a healthy diet, and the Food and Drug Administration allows "qualified health claims" for nuts and the reduction of heart disease. (More on health claims in Chapter 9.) In 2003, the FDA said that for most nuts, 1.5 ounces (43 grams) per day, as part of a diet low in saturated fat and cholesterol, "may reduce the risk of heart disease" and in 2004 that 1.5 ounces per day of walnuts as part of a diet low in saturated fat and cholesterol "may reduce the risk of coronary heart disease" as long as you don't exceed your calorie needs.

Because nuts and seeds are complex whole foods that vary—sometimes substantially—in what nutrients they contain, rather than focus on one nut or seed, enjoy a variety in the diet.

- **Almonds.** Almonds are high in monounsaturated fats, which may explain why they may help lower LDL ("bad") cholesterol levels and reduce the risk of heart disease. The antioxidant function of almond's vitamin E, along with its magnesium and potassium, may also play a role in cardiovascular health. One study found that almonds may reduce "bad" LDL cholesterol as much as statin drugs.

- **Brazil and cashew nuts.** Technically a seed, one ounce of Brazil nuts contains a whopping 774% of the daily value for selenium, and eating two Brazil nuts per day has been shown to be an effective way to increase blood levels of this antioxidant mineral. Cashew nuts are lower in fat than most nuts and contain compounds that may improve insulin sensitivity and help prevent chronic inflammation.

- **Peanuts.** Technically a legume, peanuts pack more protein per ounce than tree nuts. Want more protein and less fat? Consider powdered peanut butter. Stir it into oatmeal, yogurt, overnight oats, smoothies, protein shakes, muffin batter, salad dressings and marinades or mix it with water to create a dip for apples.

- **Pecans.** Pecans contain multiple forms of vitamin E, and are especially rich in gamma-tocopherol (one form of vitamin E), which has been shown to inhibit oxidation of LDL cholesterol. Oxidized LDL contributes to inflammation in the arteries and increse risk of cardiovascular disease. Pecans also have the highest polyphenol and flavonoid content (two types of phytonutrients) of the tree nuts.

- **Pistachios.** Studies have shown that eating in-shell pistachios enhances feelings of fullness and satisfaction while reducing caloric intake. When eating in-shell pistachios, study subjects consume about 40 percent fewer compared to already shelled pistachio kernels. Pistachios have the seconds highest polyphenol and flavonoid content of the tree nuts.

- **Walnuts.** An excellent source of the plant-based omega-3 fatty acid alpha-linolenic acid (ALA). Walnuts also boast the highest antioxidant levels of the tree nuts, followed by pecans and cashew nuts. This makes walnuts one of the best nuts for anti-inflammatory benefits. Like pecans, walnuts are unusually rich in the gamma-tocopherol form of vitamin E. The vitamin B6 found in walnuts isn't particularly plentiful, but we may absorb it particulary well. Not for nothing are walnuts shaped like a brain—eating walnuts is associated with better brain function in both younger and older adults. Walnuts are a natural source of melatonin, which is critical in the regulation of sleep, daily (circadian) rhythms and may play a role in walnuts' anti-cancer benefits.

Seeds: good nutrition in a tiny package

Why do nuts get all the nutritional glory while birds get all the seeds? Seeds offer just as much nutrition and culinary versatility as their larger cousins. Even better, they are a good dietary alternative for many people who have peanut or tree nut allergies, as allergies to edible seeds are fairly uncommon.

There's a clear difference between nuts and seeds that isn't obvious to non-botanists. My focus here is on specimens most of us think of when we think of seeds. In general, seeds are rich in the antioxidant vitamin E, which is beneficial for heart health and cancer prevention. Seeds also contain phytosterols, plant compounds that can help lower cholesterol and offer other health benefits.

- **Flaxseeds** are unique among seeds in that they are an excellent source ALA, and numerous studies have suggested that flaxseeds have cardiovascular benefits. Flaxseeds are also a good source of several nutrients, especially fiber and antioxidants. Whole flaxseeds keep for about 1-2 years in the refrigerator. Ground flaxseeds are more digestible but have a shorter shelf life, about 6-16 weeks in the refrigerator.
- **Chia seeds** have outgrown their reputation as a novelty gift item ("Ch-ch-ch-chia!") to claim status as a nutritional powerhouse. They nearly rival flaxseeds for their omega-3 and fiber content, and may help promote stable blood sugar levels after eating. These tiny seeds contain respectable amounts of calcium and other minerals important for bone health, as well as several antioxidant minerals.
- **Pumpkin seeds** are a good source of zinc, magnesium and iron. They contain small amounts of several forms of vitamin E, and research suggests that there is a health benefit to consuming E in all of its different forms. They also contain a unique blend of other antioxidant nutrients, giving them distinctive health properties. When roasting pumpkin seeds, limit oven time to 20 minutes to avoid undesirable changes to the oil inside.
- **Sunflower seeds** are a good source of many important vitamins and minerals, and are rich in the powerful antioxidant pair vitamin E and selenium. They get great ratings for phytosterol, protein and fiber content. Opt for unsalted sunflower seeds.
- **Sesame seeds** are especially rich in cholesterol-lowering phytosterols. They contain a number of minerals that are

important for bone health (such as calcium) or act as anti-oxidants (such as zinc). The unique types of fiber in sesame seeds may promote healthy blood pressure and cholesterol levels. Sesame paste (tahini) is an important ingredient in hummus. Allergies to sesame seeds are increasing, particularly among people allergic to peanuts or certain tree nuts.

Elevating the ordinary

If you really want your food to rise above "tasty" and become "delicious," you need to bust out some herbs and spices and start playing around. Why? Because when it comes to fabulous flavor, you need more than just taste, you need aroma.

When it comes to flavor, our taste buds are not particularly refined. In fact, they're pretty blunt instruments. That's because your taste buds only register the five basic tastes: sweetness, saltiness, sourness, bitterness and umami (aka, savoriness). While dishes that combine these tastes in a balanced way are pleasing to the palate, for a full flavor experience you need to add aroma.

As you've no doubt experienced, spices and herbs, as well as ingredients like grated lemon zest, are very fragrant, or aromatic. That's important, because our noses are responsible for at least 80 percent of what we perceive as flavor. Don't believe me? Try a little experiment: hold your nose and eat a jelly bean. You'll be able to tell that it's sweet, but you won't be able to tell what flavor it is. I'm sure you can also recall times when you've had a cold and found that food wasn't as appealing. If you enjoy giving dinner parties, you may have heard that it's a good idea to not use scented candles or strongly scented flowers when decorating the table, because the scent can overpower the flavor of the food.

According to Karen Page and Andrew Dornenburg, authors of the wonderful and award-winning book "The Flavor Bible," flavor is the sum total of taste + mouthfeel + aroma + the "X Factor." Mouthfeel includes temperature, texture, piquancy and astringency. The "X Factor," say Page and Dornenburg, encompasses the aspects of food that are perceived by our other senses, plus our heart, mind and spirit. More specifically:

"When we are present to what we are eating, food has the power to affect our entire selves. We experience food not only through our five physical senses—including our sense of sight, but also emotionally, mentally and spiritually."

If you've ever read the book "Like Water for Chocolate," or watched the movie version, you likely understand how flavor is about much more than what we taste and smell. (By the way, if you haven't read the book or watched the movie, I highly recommend it!)

You might be wondering how long spices keep before losing their aroma. This depends largely on the type of spice and how the spice is stored. As a general rule, whole (unground) spices keep longer than ground spices, and all spices keep longer when stored in containers with tight-fitting lids in a cool, dark cupboard. As with oils, light, heat and air are not friends of your spices.

Spices don't spoil, but they do lose their potency over time. Whole spices, stored correctly, will stay fresh for about 4 years, ground spices keep well for about 2-3 years, and dried herbs keep for 1-3 years.

Not sure how long you've had something that's sitting in your spice rack/drawer/cupboard? Rub a small amount of it in your hand then smell it and taste it. If you don't detect much aroma or flavor, then toss it and replace it.

A note on buying spices from bulk bins: While this is by far the most economical way to buy spices (spices sold in jars are very overpriced), try to buy from a store that seems to sell a lot of bulk spices. That means the turnover is likely good, and the spices they are selling are likely as fresh as possible. Bulk spices and dried herbs should also be sold from large jars with tight lids—not from the larger bulk bins used for nuts, seeds, whole grains, beans, flour and so on.

Spice it up for health

SPICES AND HERBS help make food taste great, and add delicious variety to the foods we eat. One of the major reasons that various ethnic cuisines taste different from each other is the distinctiveness offered by the herbs and spices that are traditionally used in each one.

Rosemary, oregano, basil and garlic in Italian cuisine. Cilantro, cumin and chiles in Mexican cuisine. Cardamom and curry powder in Indian cuisine. All delicious, all different.

But spices and herbs are about much more than deliciousness. They are nutritional powerhouses. Think about it for a minute: spices and herbs are plant foods. Not only can spices and herbs improve digestion and nutrient absorption, but they are concentrated sources of plant phytonutrients, many of which have antioxidant, anti-inflammatory or even anti-cancer properties. In the case of spices, these phytonutrients can be very concentrated. This is why spices like turmeric, ginger and cinnamon are heavy hitters in an anti-inflammatory diet.

- **Black Pepper.** It is probably the most popular spice in the world. Best to buy the whole peppercorns and a grinder, but buying ground is fine too. When you use turmeric,

118

use some black pepper, too, because a compound in black pepper helps your body absorb the beneficial compounds in turmeric.

- **Cinnamon.** This versatile spice can be used in both sweet and savory dishes. Add cinnamon to your breakfast oats, hot milk, cakes and pies, or meat marinades. Sprinkle it on roasted vegetables or sautéed leafy greens. Mix it into black bean dishes. Cinnamon has antioxidant and anti-inflammatory properties. Some initial studies claim it helps to reduce blood glucose and bad cholesterol, but more research is needed.
- **Garlic.** While technically a vegetable, no one eats it like a vegetable. There's no mistaking garlic when added to a dish. Freshly peeled cloves are best, but you can buy prepacked frozen minced garlic, or even garlic powder or granulated garlic
- **Ginger.** Ginger root is a cornerstone of Asian cooking, imparting a slightly sweet, slightly hot flavor. It goes well will garlic in many Thai, Indian, and Chinese dishes. You can keep a fresh ginger root in the fridge for several weeks, or in the freezer. Ground ginger powder is also an option, and you can easily sprinkle it in smoothies. Ginger has anti-inflammatory properties and may help stop nausea and may also relieve heartburn and bloating. Try a ginger and honey tea when you're under the weather.
- **Turmeric.** This bright orange powder—known to stain kitchenware—turmeric is used in Indian and other dishes for both flavor and intense color. Curcumin, the active element in turmeric, is known for healing properties such as inflammation reduction. Add turmeric to rice or add it to oil in the pan before sautéing onions and garlic. Add it to curry dishes, marinades and salad dressings. Make tea with ¼ teaspoon ground turmeric boiled in a cup of water, then strained, add honey and lemon to taste.
- **Paprika.** This bright red powder is made from ground peppers and is most associated with Hungary. Use it in stews, soups, pasta sauces, and meat dishes.
- **Oregano.** This herb, often used in Italian and Mexican cuisine, has a bold overpowering flavor, so it's best paired with strong flavored dishes.
- **Chili powder/flakes.** Most spices aren't spicy hot, but chilis are! Spicy hot food helps the body sweat and potentially re-

move toxins. Add to any dish to increase flavor and decrease the need for salt.

- **Basil.** There's nothing like a few fresh basil leaves in a tomato sauce or tomato salad. It's easy to grow basil as a potted plant on a windowsill. But even if you don't you can always find some fresh sprigs at the supermarket produce aisle. Dried leaves aren't quite the same, but it's easy to keep a jar on hand.
- **Cumin.** You can use the whole seed, but the powder is ore versatile. It is commonly used in Indian, North African and Mexican dishes. Try it sprinkled on hummus, popcorn, or pita bread with a dash of olive oil. Use it to flavor chilies, lentil soups, pork dishes, hummus and Mexican meals. Cumin is believed to help with digestion and work as an antiseptic; it is a pungent and powerful spice.
- **Allspice and Bay Leaves.** These are two separate spices, but they are often used together. Throw one bay leaf and 3-5 allspice berries into any soup, stock, or stew to increase flavor.
- **Nutmeg.** Use either the ground powder or whole nut (which needs to be grated). Nutmeg is a delicate spice to add to vegetarian dishes and creamy pasta sauces. It gives a sweet nutty aroma.

The global spice pantry

While I've got nothing against cooking from a recipe (after all, I do own a goodly amount of cookbooks), there is something to be said from being able to cook improvisationally. When you have a sense of how certain herbs, spices and other ingredients translate into certain cuisines, you are well on your way to creating tasty dishes without a recipe.

For example, when I'm craving Mexican food, I know that I can cook some beans and rice, grill some steak or chicken, sauté some peppers and onions, and season with cumin, lime juice, cilantro, salsa and hot sauce. And easy, simple, no-brainer meal that satisfies my craving.

The spices and herbs you keep in your pantry will of course depend on your favorite flavors and cuisines, as well as your comfort level with using certain spices. So your perfect spice pantry will be different than anyone else's. Here's a list of common spices for a variety of cuisines from around the world.

- **Caribbean cuisine:** Allspice, Cinnamon, Cloves, Coriander, Curry, Garlic, Gingerroot, Lime, Nutmeg, Onions, Oregano, Red Pepper, Scotch bonnet peppers and hot sauce, Thyme

- **Chinese cuisine:** Aniseed, Bean Paste, Chile Oil, Garlic, Gingerroot, Green Onions, Hot Red Peppers, Sesame Oil, Sesame Seeds, Soy Sauce, Star Anise
- **French cuisine:** Bay Leaves, Black Pepper, Chervil, Chives, Fines Herbes, Garlic, Green and Pink Peppercorns, Marjoram, Nutmeg, Onions, Parsley, Rosemary, Shallots, Tarragon, Thyme
- **German cuisine:** Allspice, Caraway Seeds, Cinnamon, Dill Seeds, Dillweed, Dry Mustard Powder, Ginger, Juniper Berries, Mustard Seeds, Nutmeg, Onions, Paprika, White Pepper
- **Greek cuisine:** Cinnamon, Dillweed, Garlic, Lemon, Mint, Nutmeg, Olives, Oregano
- **Indian cuisine:** Aniseed, Black Pepper, Cardamom Seeds, Chiles, Cilantro, Cinnamon, Cloves, Coriander Seeds, Cumin Seeds, Curry Powder, Fenugreek (an aromatic Eurasian plant used in curry powder and other spice blends), Garlic, Gingerroot, Mace, Mint, Mustard Seeds, Nutmeg, Red Pepper, Saffron, Sesame Seeds, Turmeric, Yogurt
- **Italian cuisine:** Anchovies, Basil, Bay Leaves, Fennel Seeds, Garlic, Marjoram, Onions, Oregano, Parsley, Pine Nuts, Red Pepper, Rosemary
- **Mexican cuisine:** Bell Peppers, Chiles, Cilantro, Cinnamon, Cocoa, Coriander Seeds, Cumin Seeds, Garlic, Lime, Onions, Oregano, Vanilla
- **North African cuisine:** Cilantro, Cinnamon, Coriander Seeds, Cumin Seeds, Garlic, Gingerroot, Mint, Red Pepper, Saffron, Turmeric
- **Scandinavian cuisine:** Cardamom Seeds, Dill Seeds, Dill Weed, Lemon, Mustard Seeds, Nutmeg, White Pepper
- **Spanish cuisine:** Almonds, Bell Peppers, Cumin Seeds, Garlic, Olives, Onions, Paprika, Parsley, Saffron

Chapter summary

Just as I hope Chapter 7 put lingering carb-phobia to rest, I hope that this chapter put any leftover baggage from the low-fat era out on the curb. Including healthful fats in your diet helps you enjoy your food more, especially when you start digging deeper into your spice drawer. Here are the main takeaways from Chapter 8:

Here are the main takeaways from Chapter 8:

- Not only should you not fear dietary fat, but you actually need it!
- When you put saturated fat in (dietary) context, you realize that it's the foods you eat, not isolated nutrients, that matter. That's also why just because a food is trans-fat free doesn't mean it's worth eating.
- There's a lot of misinformation about coconut oil and olive oil.
- Nuts and seeds are a great addition to your meals and snacks for nutrition health, flavor and texture.
- For food that rises above "tasty" to become "delicious," you need to play with (and even add to) the spices in your pantry.

Coming up in Chapter 9, Health Begins at Home:

- Home cooking
- Cultivating cooking skills
- What does dinner look like
- Shopping for health
- Health claims: Don't always believe what you read
- Smart food shopping

Health Begins at Home

WITH ALL THAT TALK ABOUT FLAVOR, aren't you excited to get cooking? We begin and end our days at home, so home is the place where health begins. That's why I'm a serious advocate for home cooking, and an equally serious that cooking at home doesn't have to be hard or time-consuming (unless you truly fancy yourself the next Julia Child).

In this chapter, I'll talk about:

- Why **home cooking is the key to better nutrition.**
- The bumpy, but ultimately fulfilling road to **cultivating cooking skills.**
- Why asking yourself **"What does dinner look like?"** can make it easier to answer the question "What's for dinner."
- Finally, some time- and money-saving tips for **smart food shopping.**

Home cooking: the key to better nutrition

IT'S A CURIOUS PHENOMENON that television food shows have been enjoying a robust audience for years, all while the number of daily meals cooked at home from scratch continued its gentle decline. We still eat the majority of our meals at home, but they increasingly come in the form of fast food, take-out, or heat-and-eat meals from the grocery store.

The rise of the armchair cook makes a bit more sense when you consider the program mix on The Food Network and The Cooking Channel—not to mention the runaway popularity of Bravo's Top Chef. More than half of these shows are "food-related entertainment," not "instructional cooking programs."

So, people are clearly interested in food (hey, we all eat, right), but many aren't willing to get their hands dirty in the kitchen. Don't believe me? Consumer research shows that only one-third of our main meals are cooked in the oven or on a stovetop!

Home cooking took a one-two punch last century as women began to migrate toward the workforce, and food manufacturers stepped into the fray, offering an array of "time-saving" packaged and processed foods. The marketing blitz began, whispering to women that they had better things to do than cook.

Traditionally, most women learned to cook from their mothers. So if one generation of moms ditch the kitchen, guess what happens to the cooking skills of the next generation? Most kids don't even have home economics classes to pick up the slack.

One visible fallout from this loss of basic cooking skills is a "dumbing down" of recipes in cookbooks and food magazines—a thorn in the side of those who enjoy cooking and engage in it as often as possible. It's not just the United States that is experiencing a loss of home cooks. It's happening in Europe, Japan, and quite possibly everyplace where pre-made meals are affordable and readily accessible.

So why does it matter? Why does cooking deserve to be more than just a spectator sport? Because creating and serving even the simplest of meals is a way of caring for yourself, your family, your friends. Because home-prepared meals tend to be more nutritious and lower in calories. When you cook from scratch, you know what you're eating and how much fat and salt you're adding. That may not seem important if you're healthy, but if you're managing a health condition, it makes it much easier to eat healthfully.

In pondering my ardent support of home cooking, I started thinking about why I feel so strongly that we should be preparing more of our own meals. I realized that my firm convictions are founded more on a reaction against restaurant eating than for home cooking, per se. I mean, while I do enjoy the process of cooking most of the time, sometimes it does feel like a chore and sometimes I would rather be doing something else (and then there's the dishes you have to wash afterward).

Here's my beef with restaurants: It would be very, very difficult to eat in restaurants frequently and be healthy. Not impossible, but very difficult. Basically, you would have to:

- Have enough disposable income to eat at restaurants that use fresh, local ingredients with a minimum of the pre-made soup bases and other industrially produced shortcuts that many restaurants rely on.
- Have the discernment to choose the healthiest dishes from the menu.
- Have the willpower or intuitive eating skills to stop eating before becoming overly full, no matter how much food is served to you.

Hard to do? Yes. That's why I think restaurants are best reserved as treats, not a form of daily sustenance. You know, the way it used to be in the "olden days." Even the better restaurants (with few exceptions) do not base their business model on being healthy. They base it on filling seats and selling as much food as possible. To achieve those ends, the food needs to make people want to eat more of it, in that visit and on subsequent visits. So even restaurants that use quality ingredients will likely use more fat, sugar and salt than you would at home.

There was a time when my husband and I ate in restaurants a lot. Some nice restaurants, but a lot of the "upscale casual" chain restaurants, too. And a fair amount of fast food. I've eaten at McD's once since 1999, and BK twice (and once was a salad). As the years have gone by, I've added more and more restaurants to my "never again" list, because I realize that their food is either a) kind of gross, b) overpriced for what you get or c) less satisfying than what I could make at home.

Really, other than a few favorite ethnic restaurants, an occasional jaunt to a local bakery for a scone or croissant and a few great sandwich spots I like to go to once in a blue moon, I have no love for restaurants anymore. Been there, done that, and I'm so over it. I like to know what it is I'm putting in my body, and restaurants offer too much mystery in that regard.

People who say "I can't cook" often assume that cooking is hard. Many people who can cook feel that cooking is too time consuming. Cooking can be both of those things, but it doesn't have to be.

You don't need to channel Julia Child or become an Iron Chef to roast a few chicken breasts and potatoes and toss a salad. There's very little prep work, and while you keep a casual eye on things, you have time to check the mail, unload the dishwasher, feed the dog, and so on. That's what I often find myself doing!

Even the most fledgling of home cooks can do amazing things by learning a few core skills. One or two ways to cook vegetables. How to make a simple vinaigrette. How to cook a pot of rice. What to do with a piece of meat or fish (or block of tofu, if you prefer). You don't need to be adept at following a recipe or know any complicated kitchen techniques. Nail down a few basics, assemble a small collection of condiments and seasonings that appeal to your taste buds, and you're golden.

Cultivating cooking skills

WHEN I WAS TEACHING MYSELF TO COOK in my first college apartment, there were tears on more than one occasion. I have vivid memories of crying, "Dinner's RUINED!" after an unfortunate experiment with green bean stroganoff (read: curdled yogurt) out of *Laurel's Kitchen* (my first cookbook purchase, now slightly tattered but still on my bookshelves).

It's an amazing thing to take a handful of ingredients and turn them into a tasty, healthy dish. It's like alchemy. (OK, occasionally it's a disaster, but usually it's like alchemy.) And even the occasional disaster isn't really the end of the world, unless you're playing with really expensive ingredients. For years I didn't know how to cook beef or pork, partly because I was a near-vegetarian when I was learning to cook, and also because meat can be expensive, and I was afraid to screw it up. The fear of messing up beans and rice doesn't seem to carry the same weight.

My mother worked (not always full-time) and she cooked (not fancy French meals or anything). So I grew up being exposed to home cooking, even though I don't recall ever really helping out in the kitchen (other than when it was cookie-baking time). More than once in our married life, my husband has said to me, half-jokingly, "Didn't your mother teach you anything?" No, not really. I did a little cooking in high school, when it was just me and my dad, but that was mostly limited to Shake n' Bake chicken and boxed rice or noodle mixes. And spaghetti...I could make a decent spaghetti with red sauce even then. And pork chops with apples and onions.

So, I entered into adulthood with the idea that dinner did not come from a drive-thru window and that it did involve vegetables, but lacked the skills to confidently assemble a meal. I'm pretty much self-taught. In the beginning, there were more disasters, less alchemy, but with the wisdom of hindsight I can see that I aimed too high some of the time.

Anyway, despite that fact that my early attempts to expand my cooking skills were rocky at times, but I persevered, because I knew it was a worthwhile venture. Today, I love to cook, and am not afraid to tackle complicated recipes, provided I have adequate time and space. (I also embrace the idea that cooking is kind of like a science experiment: sometimes you're not going to get the results you hoped for, and that's all part of the learning process.)

When time is in short supply, I know I can lean heavily on the most basic of cooking skills to still put healthy food on my dinner table and in my lunchbag, without resorting to takeout. I eat a LOT of baked chicken breasts, green salads and roasted vegetables (often in the same meal). I never really get tired of them, especially because they are such versatile items. They are the kitchen what the little black dress is to the clothes closet (for women, anyway). You can find these "little black dress" recipes in the recipe section at the end of the book.

What does dinner look like?

EVEN THOUGH MANY OF US cook and eat on the fly, at least some of the time, the June Cleaver-era idea of what dinner looks like still manages to linger in our consciousness. A roast, potatoes, two vegetables, dinner rolls, dessert. I love a good roast as much as the next person, but that's an occasional weekend meal...not a weeknight staple (although the leftovers might be!).

Some new vegetarians have a hard time breaking free of the notion of meat at the center of the plate, with side dishes as the supporting players. I think it's a similar mindset when you're really busy, but you want to prepare a healthy dinner for yourself or your family. "How am I going to cook a proper entree and side dishes when it's 6 p.m. and everyone's starving?"

I can count on three fingers the weeknights when I have a "proper" entree and side dishes on my table. Other nights, I am much more liberal in my interpretation of dinner, provide it follows three simple rules. It must include:

- Abundant vegetables
- A serving of healthy protein
- A touch of healthy fat

Grains or starchy vegetables are optional, and primarily depend on how many carbohydrate-rich foods I had at breakfast and lunch and how hungry I am. Don't forget, vegetables offer some healthy carbs, too, full of fiber and richer in nutrients.

Eggs are a favorite. They aren't just for breakfast anymore! It takes about a minute to wilt some spinach, kale or other greens in a pan with a little olive oil. Add the eggs, scramble, add some salt and pepper and a little feta or Parmesan cheese, and you've got dinner. I always have mixed salad greens on hand, so while I keep one eye on the eggs, I can focus the other on tossing a quick salad.

Speaking of salads...I eat a lot of salads. Big, main-dish salads. Tossed with homemade vinaigrette, topped with cherry tomatoes, chunks of bell pepper or cucumbers (I try to pre-chop a few and keep them in the fridge) or leftover roasted vegetables. For protein, I'll add leftover chicken or steak, if I have it, or a big dollop of hummus. Or a veggie burger patty. For the healthy fat, I'll add avocado or walnuts (if I need some grains, I'll often toast a piece of sprouted grain bread and use the avocado as a spread). I may add a touch of blue or feta cheese.

Soup and a salad. A tuna or turkey sandwich and a salad. Fish sticks (high-quality ones, please) on a bed of shredded cabbage topped with salsa, avocado, sour cream or plain Greek yogurt, and maybe a touch of shredded cheddar cheese. Or swap canned beans and leftover rice for the fish sticks. You get the idea...and I'm sure you'll come up with you own ideas!

What I won't do is eat cereal for dinner, mostly because I am so busy that I don't even want to start down that road, because it might become a crutch. The only frozen "convenience" foods I keep in the house are veggie burgers, fish sticks, broccoli, and occasionally some ravioli. And yet I feed myself healthfully and well every night...even when I am so busy I think my head might explode. Where there's a will, there's a way...that's all I'm saying.

Smart food shopping

IF YOU'RE GOING TO EAT, and you're not going to rely on other people to prepare your food for you, then you need to grocery shop. When you have a smart shopping strategy, not only will you make healthier, more nutritious choices, but you'll save time and money!

Shop less often. Has a trip to the grocery store become a daily activity? Shopping once a week instead of once a day can save you hours of time driving, parking, and waiting in line, and it will also cut down on "impulse purchases" which tend to be less healthy items (they also make up about 40 percent of the average shopper's grocery bill). If you plan ahead, and make good use of your freezer, you can trim your food shopping to once a week or even less. (I'll talk all about meal planning in Chapter 11.)

Buy in bulk. Most natural food stores, and more and more supermarkets, now have bulk bins. You can often save more than 30 percent on the cost of food by buying in bulk rather than purchasing prepackaged items. Whole grains, legumes (beans, lentils, dried peas), nuts and seeds, dried fruit and spices and seasonings are just some of the foods that are often available in bulk bins. When you shop in bulk, you can buy as much or as little as you need, which helps reduce food waste.

Consider pre-cut veggies. Buying these may cost a bit more money, but can also save time.

Choose convenience foods wisely. There are many ready-to-eat foods that have sacrificed good nutrition in order to be convenient. They may have added vitamins and bill themselves as nutritional superstars, but actually be nearly void of real nutritional value. Other ready-to-eat foods are nearly the equal of home cooked, and represent legitimate ways to save time without sacrificing health. Paying attention to the Nutrition Facts panel and ignoring the marketing hype on the front of the package can help you choose those convenience foods that are actually good for you.

Don't shop hungry. Do I have to explain why? When you're hungry, those cookies or that ice cream is more likely to just hop into your cart ("How did that get in there?"), even if you are shopping with a list...

Shop with a list. It helps you reduce impulse purchases (which tends to be good for your wallet and your health, because most people don't buy broccoli on impulse) and, when you organize your list by category (produce, bulk bins, dairy, etc.) can help you get in and out of the store faster. It also helps reduce the odds that you will have to run back to the store later to pick up a forgotten ingredient. Of course, a smart list comes from smart meal planning, which I will talk all about in Chapter 11.

Chapter summary

When eating nutritious food is important to you, knowing how to shop, and how to cook (even if it's simple cooking) are two formidable tools in your toolbox.

Here are the main takeaways from Chapter 9:

- Home cooking is a way to care for yourself (and friends and family) in a deeply meaningful way.
- Cultivating cooking skills doesn't mean becoming a gourmet cook, but it does mean that you will be be able to feed yourself well.
- The answer to "What does dinner look like?" doesn't have to be complicated.
- How smart food shopping can save you valuable time that would be better spent actually preparing a meal!

Coming up in Chapter 10, Your Eating Day:

- Meal timing and spacing
- Smart snacking
- Grazing

PART 3

When

"First we eat, then we do everything else."
– M.F.K. FISHER

Your Eating Day

EVEN THE MOST NUTRITIOUS diet is missing something if you eat at irregular times, dine when you're distracted, or snack because you're stressed or bored. While there is no clear, consistent evidence about when or how often we should eat, for weight or health, skipping meals, eating on the run and grazing are a few habits that don't do us any favors. Other than that, your ideal eating pattern will be unique to you.

In this chapter, I'll talk about:

- Why your **meal timing and spacing** matters, but there's no one formula that works for everyone.
- Why **smart snacking** can be a tool for managing hunger and fitting extra nutrition into your day.
- Why nibbling or **grazing** your way through the day isn't an optimal way to eat.
- And, a **lunch break manifesto.**

135

Meal timing & spacing

EATING FOR HEALTH isn't just about what you eat, it's about when, why and how you eat. Let's start with the when. We make numerous eating choices over the course of a day: What to eat, why to eat, where to eat, how to eat and finally when to eat. When you're trying to eat healthfully, it's common to search for that missing detail that might provide the key to perfect health and your desired weight.

Optimal meal timing and frequency, otherwise known as when and how often to eat, is one holy grail. Are there best and worst times of day to eat? Is there a "right" number of meals to eat each day? Is grazing a better way to eat…or does our gut need downtime between "eating events"? As with many questions about food and nutrition, the answer is, "It depends." While there are many opinions, expert and otherwise, about the optimal number of daily meals and snacks, there is no clear, consistent evidence that links meal timing or frequency with your weight or your health.

Eating more frequently is sometimes associated with excess body weight and lower nutrition, sometimes not. Skipping meals is sometimes linked to higher weights or poor health…but sometimes it isn't. Eating more often can help manage hunger, or more meals may simply mean more calories. Eating late at night can be a problem, but generally only if it interferes with sleep or results in extra calories (although there are good reasons to avoid night eating whenever possible, which I talk about below).

Some research suggests that snacking causes weight gain, while other research suggests that avoiding snacking causes weight gain (more on snacking in a few pages). One study randomly assigned individuals to either eat three meals each day, or three meals plus three snacks. Everyone ate the same number of calories. There were no notable differences in weight loss or measurements of appetite between the two eating styles.

Some people skip meals in an attempt to cut calories, others to save time ("I'm just too busy to stop and eat lunch."). Many meal skippers claim to not be hungry at certain times of the day, most commonly at breakfast or lunch. Often, the hunger is there, but we don't notice it because our mornings are chaotic, or we've made such a habit of ignoring mid-day hunger when we're busy that we lose the ability to recognize it.

What does this mean for you? It means that what you eat probably makes more of a difference than how often you eat. If you are making healthful food choices, eating to meet your body's energy needs, and your hunger rarely flares out of control, then worrying about when and how often you eat is splitting hairs.

If you do feel like your food habits could use a tune up, start by examining whether your food choices support good nutrition. When you eat breakfast, lunch and dinner, you typically choose different foods at each meal, so skipping meals can make it harder to get the variety of foods and nutrients you need for good health. Snacking can be a good opportunity to add extra servings of fruits, vegetables, whole grains and protein into you day, or it can be an opportunity to eat foods that offer little in the way of nutrition.

Your ideal meal frequency will give you steady energy throughout the day and let you get hungry enough between meals that you feel ready to eat a nourishing meal but not so hungry that you are ready to eat the first thing you lay eyes on (aka "hijack" hunger or "primal" hunger). Ask yourself these questions:

- What are my hunger levels like during the day?
- Do I get ravenous between meals?
- Do I even feel actual physical hunger?
- How are my energy levels? (Note, poor sleep also contributes to low energy.)

If you feel ravenous between meals, that's a sign that you need to eat more at your meals (possibly just more protein), or that you need to eat more often. If you realize that you rarely experience true hunger, or feel stuffed rather than simply satisfied after you eat, you may need to eat a little less at meals, or eat less often.

For many people, three meals + a healthy afternoon snack (say, fruit and nuts) can give adequate space between meals to "rest and digest" while not allowing hunger to get "primal." This is especially true when we work away from home, because the space between lunch and dinner is often long enough for hunger to get the upper hand without an afternoon snack. Generally speaking, this type of meal spacing promotes nice, stable blood sugar levels, especially when coupled with healthy food choices.

Intermittent fasting and "eating windows"

You might wonder about intermittent fasting (IF). Certainly, there's been a lot written about it in the last several years, and you won't find a shortage of books (electronic or traditionally published) extolling its benefits for both weight loss and improvements in metabolic parameters (blood sugar, blood lipids, inflammation) that contribute to type 2 diabetes, heart disease and cancer.

Trouble is, there's not a lot of scientific research to back up those claims! In fact, most research data comes from animal studies (and you are not a lab rat). Much of the human data comes from observing participants of religious-based fasts (such as Ramadan), or from experimental studies that are too small and brief to provide meaningful information.

In today's diet culture, IF takes on a few different forms. **Alternate-day fasting** involves eating nothing one day, but eating what you want (of healthy foods, hopefully) the next. Then repeat, repeat. **Modified fasting** is similar, but on fasting days individuals eat about ¼ of what they would normally eat. **Time-restricted feeding** narrows the day's "eating window" to anywhere from 8-12 hours.

The best information we have is about the third form of "fasting," not necessarily because the research studies are any better (they still rely heavily on lab rodents), but because there are known benefits to limiting our eating to daytime, and they mostly have to do with staying in sync with our circadian rhythms.

In a nutshell, we have two biologic clocks. Our "master" clock lives in our brain and responds to light and dark. We also have a "peripheral" clock (housed in the liver and other body tissues) that primarily responds to food. We evolved to restrict our activity (including eating) to daytime, so when we eat at night, our master clock and peripheral clock become out of sync.

I strongly discourage meal skipping (of the unintentional fasting or "whoops, I was too busy to eat" variety) in anyone who has trouble wrangling their hunger when they next eat (or in anyone who needs to eat on a regular basis due to specific medication schedules or health issues). But I do encourage honoring at least a 12-hour "fasting window" overnight. Part of this is for biological reasons (you don't want your body clocks to get desynchronized, do you?). Part of this is purely practical.

For individuals who struggle with eating for non-hunger reasons (stress, emotions, boredom) with or without overt cravings, the period between dinner and bedtime can be tricky. The food consumed during this time tends to be of the snacky/salty/sugary variety, and may also involve grazing. Making it a practice to honor an overnight fasting window (one that's longer than the hours you spend sleeping) can help you avoid mindlessly eating food your body doesn't need. Unless you have an evening medication dose that must be taken with food, or your doctor or dietitian has advised you to have a bedtime snack due to blood sugar issues, there's no reason to eat in the late evening if your dinner was nutritious and adequately portioned, and if you have a nutritious breakfast planned to "break your fast"! Of course, if you ate a light or early dinner and feel genuinely hungry before bedtime, and that hunger will keep you awake, then a light-but-nourishing snack is probably called for!

Smart snacking

ASK A DOZEN PEOPLE what they think of snacking, and you'll likely get a dozen answers. It ruins your appetite. It helps you avoid getting too hungry between meals. It's a great way to fit more veggies into your day. It's an excuse to eat candy and chips. It helps you avoid weight gain. It makes you gain weight. It's a nice little fuel break in your day. It's something to help pass the time while you watch TV.

Each of these answers are part of the snacking habits of average Americans—for better or for worse. Research has identified two major types of snackers:

- Individuals who snack several times a day in response to true hunger. This type of snacking, which likely happens at regular times, allows adjustment of food intake from day to day, depending on the body's needs.
- Individuals who choose snacks high in salt, sugar or fat and tend to snack at irregular times in response to environmental stimuli—not because of hunger. Snacking while watching TV is common. This type of snacking is not in response to the body's needs, and tends to lead to poor nutrition.

According to data from the National Health and Nutrition Examination Survey (NHANES), in the early 1970s, the average man got 502 of his daily calories from snacks, the average woman got 296. Jump forward 40 years, and those numbers increase to 634 calories for men and 438 for women. Today, fewer Americans eat three meals a day, but most of us snack. In fact, 2 out of 3 Americans eat two or more snacks each day. We get about 23 percent of our calories from snacks—that's twice the average calories eaten at breakfast and about the same as the average lunch calories.

When are we doing this snacking? If you tend to eat both lunch and dinner, there's a 2 in 3 chance that you eat a snack in between, and a similar chance that you eat a snack between dinner and bedtime. Only about 1 in 3 of us snack between breakfast and lunch.

It's true that many snack foods and beverages are high in fat, salt, sugar and refined grains, providing extra calories but minimal nutrition. However, NHANES data suggests that our snacks are often more nutritious than that, with common snack foods including fruit, nuts, seeds, whole grains and milk.

Snacking can either work for you, or against you. Considering that snacks are making up more and more of our daily calories, it's worth understanding how to snack smartly:

- Smart snackers use snacks to include more nutrition in their day, combining some quality carbohydrates with a little protein and fat for staying power. For example, an apple and a small handful of nuts, Greek yogurt and berries, raw veggies and hummus. Use well-timed snacks to take the edge off their hunger so they aren't ravenous when their next meal comes.
- Not-so-smart snackers choose high-calorie, high-carb, nutrient-poor foods, eat whether or not they are hungry, often grazing on whatever's available. As I mentioned, excessive snacking/grazing makes it hard to feel true hunger.

Do your snacking habits need a tune up?

Keep a food log for a week or two—you may be surprised at what you learn! If you find you're snacking when you're not hungry, exploring the reasons why (food availability, boredom, stress, cravings) is a good idea. If you find that you are truly hungry enough for a snack between meals, make sure you have nourishing foods on hand so you aren't running to the vending machine, coffee shop or convenience store.

Grazing

WHILE MANY PEOPLE find that they feel best with three meals and two snacks (one between breakfast and lunch, one between lunch and dinner), I encourage my patients to be cautious about slipping into a grazing eating pattern. When you graze, you eat so frequently that you might never feel true hunger, and you don't eat enough at any one time to feel true satiety/fullness. This makes it difficult to eat intuitively or mindfully. Additionally, we simply don't have a good sense of how much we eat in the course of a day when our food comes in a scattered stream of bites and nibbles.

Grazing can take on many forms. It could mean eating a little here, a little there, throughout the day, either because you don't have (or don't feel that you have) time to eat a proper lunch at work or because you don't feel like taking the time to make yourself real meals when you're at home. Or, it might mean not allowing yourself enough food to be satisfied at meals, so you end up nibbling from your kitchen or work break room.

Even when you eat an adequate portion of a proper meal, if you ate mindlessly and barely noticed your food, you may feel the need to keep nibbling and grazing, even though you aren't technically hungry.

If you're on child-feeding or dinner-dish-cleanup duty, you may end up nibbling on the food your child wouldn't eat, or those little bit of left-over food in the pan, "Because there's not enough to save and it would be a shame to waste it."

If you're already hungry when you're preparing dinner, you may find yourself nibbling and noshing to the point where you aren't hungry any-more when the meal you took time to prepare is ready to eat!

If you tend to graze, ask yourself why.
- Are you not setting boundaries in a busy schedule (every-one deserves a lunch break)?
- Do you feel, consciously or possibly subconsciously, that you don't deserve to eat a full meal (this can be a hold over from the dieting mentality).
- Are you constantly eating because you're afraid of feeling hungry?

The fact is that each of needs to eat real meals spaced across our day, possibly with snacks. And it's a good thing to feel gentle hunger. Sensa-tions of hunger and fullness are our internal guides of when and how much to eat.

A lunch break manifesto

WHEN DID TAKING A LUNCH BREAK become a bad thing? If I had a nickel for every patient who doesn't take a proper lunch break, I'd be able to take myself out to lunch. I'm not just talking about people who work outside the home—I have many a retiree, telecommuter or stay-at-home parent who doesn't grant themselves the time to sit down midday and eat some-thing resembling an actual meal. The reasons vary, but the outcomes are similar—and those outcomes may not be good.

I frequently see three less-than-ideal lunch behaviors. One is skipping lunch altogether. The second is hastily wolfing down lunch while working or engaged in another activity. The third is half-heartedly grabbing some sort of snack—possibly even scavenged from the break room or a desk drawer—instead of an actual meal. There are even more reasons why this happens:
- Occupations where taking a break midday is challenging,

such as retail or restaurant jobs.
- Work meetings scheduled during the lunch hour.
- A boss/manager/employer who frowns on people being gone from their desk for more than five minutes (unless it's because they're in a meeting).
- A work culture in which employees treat coworkers like slackers if they take a lunch break.
- Self-imposed notions about working through lunch being a badge of honor, or that you don't deserve to take a measly half-hour for yourself (never mind a full lunch hour).
- The fear that if you take a lunch break, your job will be out-sourced to a robot.

I have tech and aerospace employees who only have time to eat while walking from a meeting in one building to another meeting in another building. I have government employees who would get the stink eye if they left the office to eat their lunch. I have teachers and lawyers who skip both breakfast and lunch because they "don't have time." I have retirees, stay-at-home parents and telecommuters who don't stop what they're doing in order to eat lunch, then wonder why they're raiding the kitchen at 3 p.m.

This problem starts early. According to a 2015 report by the University of Washington Nutritional Sciences program and the Seattle Public School District Nutrition Task Force, elementary schools students in Seattle Public Schools spend about 13 minutes eating lunch, resulting in a lot of food waste (especially of fruits and vegetables, which take longer to eat). This sets up unhealthy habits that can persist for life.

Skipping—or scrimping on—meals can lead to overeating later on when steadily growing hunger reaches primal levels. Regularly neglecting the very real physiological need to eat something mid-day can make it very difficult to recognize "normal" hunger cues, and can even kill off those signals over time. When I have patients with dead hunger signals, it's almost always due to a long-standing habit of skipping lunch (and sometimes breakfast). Why should your body keep telling you it's hungry if you never listen?

I say it's time to take back lunch. Instead of stoically working through the lunch hour, eat your lunch (away from your desk, ideally), then go for a short walk, or meditate, or people watch, or run an errand, or start learning a new language (there are apps for that). If you are an employer or manager who cultivates a work culture that discourages taking time for a proper lunch, you're doing your business a disservice. Employees who take lunch breaks are happier, healthier—and more productive. Just some food for thought.

Chapter summary

I hope that this chapter eases any anxiety you may have had about how often to eat, and helps you see the value of cultivating intuitive and mindful eating skills to guide your eating.

Here are the main takeaways from Chapter 10:

- There's no magic number of meals/snacks to eat and no universally perfect timing for health and nutrition.
- Smart snacking can be a great way to manage hunger and add extra nutrition to your day, or not-so-smart snacking can be a way to add excess calories (often mindlessly).
- Grazing your way through the day isn't a ticket to satisfying eating.
- Eat lunch!

Coming up in Chapter 11, Finding The Time:

- Meal planning 101
- Planning a perfect pantry
- Meals in minutes
- Too busy to eat well?

Finding the Time

WHETHER YOU'RE COOKING for a family of four or five in the suburbs, preparing meals for one or two in a small city kitchen, or feeding an extended family in the country, everyone needs to eat. Generally speaking, meals prepared at home are going to be more healthful and less expensive than meals purchased outside the home, especially when you have a strategy for the week's meals.

In this chapter, I'll talk about:

- How investing a little time in **meal planning** can pay off in spades, saving you both time and stress and supporting better nutrition.
- Why **planning a perfect pantry** will save you time when grocery shopping (and even save your bacon when you haven't had time to grocery shop).
- How to put together **meals in minutes** by staying organized.
- Why thinking you're **too busy to eat well** is usually not the case...even when you are truly busy.

Meal planning 101

MOST OF THE STRESS of cooking comes from arriving home late, with no clear idea of exactly what ingredients you have that you can use to cook. By creating a dinner plan for the week, you eliminate all that stress. You know what you're planning to cook, and you know you'll have all the ingredients on hand.

Planning gets a bad rap as being boring and time-consuming. But when develop the habit of investing some up-front time to make a meal plan for the week, you'll find that it quickly become routine and ends up saving you both time and money, because you avoid last minute dashes to the supermarket and also avoid buying ingredients you forgot you already had in your pantry.

So what does it take to become a savvy, organized meal planner and grocery shopper?

Habit 1: Stock your kitchen with staples. A "staple" is whatever you need to make the kind of food you like to cook. For many people, pasta is a staple, or canned tuna. For others, soy sauce or anchovy paste might be must-have foods. With a well-stocked pantry, you can make many of your favorite dishes any day of the week without stopping again at the market. You will also have the luxury of purchasing pantry staples when they are on sale, instead of the moment you need them for a specific dish.

Habit 2: Space allowing, back up your staples. Buy and store one more of each staple if you have space, keeping you from dashing to the market at the last minute for just a single essential ingredient. It's like having your own private store at your fingertips!

Habit 3: Keep a running grocery list. Tuck a long skinny pad into the front of your silverware drawer, clip a sheet of paper to the fridge with a magnet, or keep a list in your mobile device, and try to add things to your grocery list throughout the week, as you think of them. Do a quick inventory of your pantry and fridge before you go to the store—you may find last minute omissions, or get ideas of what to buy to pair with other foods on hand.

Habit 4: Plan a week's worth of meals (see "Meal Planning Basics," below). This is the step most people resist: planning the week's meals. Write the days of the week on a piece of paper, and jot down your dinner plan for each day. At first it might take you a half hour, but you'll pare that down to 10 minutes or so once you get in the habit. (Hot tip: there's nothing wrong with making one plan, then using that same plan every week. Or make two plans and just alternate them, week by week. You're the cook. If someone else wants more variety, let them volunteer to cook!)

Most of the stress of cooking comes from arriving home late, with no clear idea of exactly what ingredients you have that you can use to cook. By creating a dinner plan for the week, you eliminate all that stress. You know what you're planning to cook, and you know you'll have all the ingredients on hand.

Habit 5: Make a shopping list. Once you know what you'll be eating for dinner each day, add any additional dinner ingredients or pantry staples to your existing running grocery list. Then, think about lunch, and breakfast, and add any routine ingredients for those meals. Now your list is complete and it's time to go to the store!

Habit 6: Shop intentionally. Armed with your list, you should be able to shop fairly quickly. At the start of each aisle, glance at your list and note which items you'll find in that aisle. (Some people even like to organize their list by aisle so they are less likely to forget something.) Try to buy only what's on your list, and limit impulse items to a minimum. Note: Resisting impulse items is easier if you don't shop on an empty stomach!

Habit 7: Store food thoughtfully. Before you put away your food, clean out anything in the fridge that's on its last legs.

Toss the leftover containers with three bites of moldy green beans, or the carton with an inch of sour milk. Make a pile of tired veggies you can turn into a zesty stir-fry or add to a pot of chili tonight. Rearrange what's left, and only then put away your new purchases. Pantry items such as crackers, pita chips, and cereal can go stale quickly after opening, increasing the risk of food waste. Try using large binder clips (much less expensive than "chip clips") to keep the bag closed. You can also use gallon-size Ziplock-type bags, and reuse them for similar types of foods. If you have room, freeze extras of foods that have oil content to avoid rancidity. These include whole wheat and whole grain flours, nuts, and butter. Store olive and other cooking oils in a dark place, and refrigerate cooking vinegars to ensure optimum freshness.

Habit 8: Prep food ahead of time. There's one more step after you return home and unpack your food: prepping fruits and veggies, especially greens, and putting them away in appropriate containers. This extends extend the shelf life of your purchases, and make it easy to grab healthy foods quickly.

- Slice up a melon.
- Wash and spin-dry lettuce or other leafy greens.
- Cut up carrot and celery sticks.
- Chop veggies, such as cucumbers and bell peppers, for a few days of salads.

146

Meal planning basics

Decide what day(s) work best for grocery shopping, and then back up from there to decide when to do your meal planning. For example, if you do your primary shopping on, say, Saturday morning, you may want to do your planning on Thursday or Friday. If you like to choose new recipes to try, this gives you the earlier part of the week to browse your favorite recipe sources.

The plan

Print out the Weekly Meal Planner or the Detailed Weekly Meal Planner from the website (or simply write the days of the week on a piece of paper):

- Look at your schedule. Do you have planned meals out?
  Are guests coming over for dinner? Note this on your plan.
  Next, ask yourself (and answer) these two questions:
- How often am I willing to cook?
- How high is my (or my family's) tolerance for leftovers?

If you don't want to cook very often during the week, but love (or don't mind) leftovers, then you can plan to cook or prepare larger portions of food less often (i.e. batch cooking). If you don't like leftovers but want to prepare more meals at home, then choose recipes that fit within your time and energy parameters. Most nights of the week, simple is best.

New to you, or tried-and-true?

If you love picking out new recipes to try each week, then carve out some time to browse cookbooks, magazines, food blogs or recipe sites, and plug what excites you into your plan. Otherwise, consider developing a sort of "meal template." To do this, start by identifying which types of meals you eat most often? For example:

- Big salads
- Meat/Poultry + veggies
- Fish + veggies
- Pasta/grain dishes
- Beans/lentils
- Soups
- Quick meals (scrambled eggs, quesadillas, tacos, etc.)

Based on how often you want to cook each week, divvy up your main meal categories. If you have more categories than "cooking nights," you may want to combine some categories. (i.e., Wednesday is either a big salad night or a soup night). Two tips for making the most of this sort of "template" plan:

- There's nothing wrong with using the same plan every week (Tuesday may be "Taco Tuesday" but you can have fish tacos one week, chicken tacos the next, and so on). Or make two plans and just alternate them, week by week. You're the cook. If someone else wants more variety, let them volunteer to cook!
- Collect some fail safe recipes for each category. Keep copies in a folder or slim binder that you use for your regular weeknight meals.

Next, decide how many servings you need to prepare on each cooking night, based on how many servings of leftovers you need for additional dinners and lunches, or whether you want to freeze some leftovers for future meals. Add any ingredients you need to buy to your shopping list.

Once you know what you'll be eating for dinner each day, think about lunch and breakfast (factoring in any planned meals out or available leftovers). Often, this is as simple as "I'm going to alternate between scrambled eggs with veggies + toast and Greek yogurt with berries + walnuts for breakfast this week," and "On days I don't have leftovers, I'll have a sandwich or salad for lunch" and add any routine ingredients for those meals.

More planning tips

Keep a sheet of paper on the side of your fridge, or keep a list in your mobile device, and try to add things to your grocery list throughout the week, as you think of them. This includes pantry staples like rice and spices, as well as perishable items that you use regularly, but not necessarily for specific recipes, such as eggs or Greek yogurt.

Do a quick inventory of your pantry and fridge before you go to the store—you may find last minute omissions, or get ideas of what to buy to pair with other foods on hand.

Even if you enjoy experimenting with new recipes, it's helpful to type up a list (on your phone or elsewhere) of quick meals as reminders of what to make when you are extra busy or just don't feel like cooking. Quick meals could include picking up a rotisserie chicken and tossing a green salad for the side, or, in the immortal words of the legendary food writer and cookbook author Elizabeth David, an omelette and a glass of wine (preferably with a salad on the side).

Preventing food waste

No one likes food waste. When you find yourself throwing away food that you spent good money on (even if you have a robust food budget), guilt often comes along for the ride. Making a weekly meal plan, along with proper storage and advance prep, will help keep food waste to a minimum.

Final thoughts

Getting into the habit of meal planning is, like any other habit, something you have to cultivate. It may feel like it takes too much time at first, but it becomes faster and more routine as you go along. Remember that there's no one right way to do it, but doing it makes it easier to achieve any nutrition and health goals you have for yourself, plus it can put an end to that tedious end-of-the-day question, "What's for Dinner?"

Planning a perfect pantry

IF I HAD TO SHOP every week for everything I eat in that week, I think I would go insane. Even in my perfect ideal world where I have lots of time to cook and plan meals in advance (a world I don't currently inhabit, alas), I would still enjoy being able to "shop" my pantry. It's much easier to stock up on non-perishable items you use often when your supplies are a bit low than it is to buy every item individually each time you need it.

I keep a magnetic notepad on the side of my refrigerator. When I notice I'm about to run out of coffee, oatmeal, rice, canned beans, mineral water, spices or whatnot, I write it down, if I don't have my smartphone, and it's "Reminders" app, handy. Then on my weekly shopping trip, I buy those few items, plus enough fresh produce, milk and yogurt for the week (I add eggs when my hens aren't laying). Very streamlined, which is what I need right now with my hectic life! My pantry is so well stocked that many weeks, the perishable items are all that's on my list.

If you like to keep a pantry (not everyone does, but I really do recommend it), stocking it with YOUR staples items is another great way to save yourself time and money. Here are a few tips:

- A "staple" is whatever you need to make the kind of food you like to cook. For many people, pasta is a staple, or canned tuna. For others, soy sauce or anchovy paste might be must-have foods.

- With a well-stocked pantry, you can make many of your favorite dishes any day of the week without stopping again at the market. You will also have the luxury of purchasing pantry staples when they are on sale, instead of the moment you need them for a specific dish.
- Buy and store extras of each staple if you have space, and then add it to your shopping list when you start to run a bit low.

So what's in the Perfect Pantry? That depends on you! Here are some of my go-to items:

Pantry

- Canned tuna and salmon
- Whole grains (brown, red, black and wild rices; various forms of whole wheat, such as farro and bulgur, quinoa, polenta, sorghum)
- Pasta (although I don't eat it often)
- Oatmeal and other multi-grain hot cereals
- Canned beans (white, pinto, black and chickpeas)
  Dry beans (for when I have the time and forethought to cook them)
- Canned tomatoes (diced, sauce, paste, and sometimes whole and crushed)
- Canned artichoke hearts
- Jarred roasted red peppers
- Canned green chilis
- Organic tomato or tomato-red pepper soup
- Chicken broth (in cans or cartons)
- Almond milk (for smoothies)
- Dried fruits (to use in oatmeal)
- Assorted vinegars (red, white, cider, balsamic, sherry, rice)
- Extra virgin olive oil (one for cooking, a nicer one for salads)
- Avocado oil
- Hot sauces
- Spices

Refrigerator

- Capers
- Kalamata olives
    n and other good mustards
    nut and hazelnut oils (for salads, NOT for cooking!)

- Quality mayonnaise (which I don't use often)
- Plain Greek yogurt
- Milk
- A few cheeses (Parmesan, blue, feta)
- Salad greens
- Fruit for snacks
- Lemons and limes
- Other seasonal produce
- Peanut and almond butters

Freezer

- Raw nuts (walnuts, almonds and pecans)
- Whole grain flour
- Sprouted grain bread (and sometimes English muffins or pita bread)
- Veggie burgers
- Chicken breasts and thighs
- At least one whole chicken
- Salmon fillets
- Frozen berries (for smoothies)
- Beef (we buy 1/4 of a steer every year from a local small farm)
- Containers of leftover soups and stews
- Homemade chicken and beef broth

Meals in minutes

DO YOU THINK HEALTHY EATING and cooking require hours in the kitchen? Many people say their main barriers to healthy eating are time, money, lack of motivation and lack of knowledge. I can't help you with the money part, and hopefully you've already dug deep and found your motivation, but I can give you some tips to help with the time issue. (Sometimes, time is money!) Here are some tips that will help you make healthy, satisfying meals in minutes:

Keep your pantry or cupboard stocked. If I haven't mentioned this enough, with a fully-stocked pantry or cupboard, it's a snap to make a healthy meal quickly.

Be organized. Restaurant chefs have to be organized. It's helpful for home cooks, too. Chefs call it mise en place, a French phrase that means "putting in place," (as in setting up). You'll happily find you can save time in the long run if you prep all ingredients—or make your own mise en place—before you start cooking. Cleaning as you cook will minimize after meal cleanup.

Don't peel your produce. The healthiest diets, including anti-inflammatory and Mediterranean-style diets, feature plenty of vegetables. You'll save time if you skip the peeling whenever possible. Instead, wash produce thoroughly and get the extra fiber and nutrients in the skins.

Consider canned and frozen. Find healthy convenience foods, like canned beans, canned or pouched tuna, frozen vegetables or canned and jarred tomatoes, and use them as the base for a healthy meal. Match them with other ingredients such as whole grains, spices and herbs or marry a canned version with a frozen ingredient for an extra fast and healthy meal. Fresh isn't the only option.

Cook batches of whole grains ahead of time. Whole grains are a perfect foundation for delicious Mediterranean meals. Pick your favorite whole grain(s), cook large batches and freeze for future meals.

Cook one thing and use it in many ways. For example, roast a chicken on the weekend and use the meat in meals throughout the week:

- Sliced and served hot immediately after roasting
- Topping a green salad for lunch the next day
- Mixed with pasta or rice and a vegetable
- Make soup.

Another example: grill a few sliced eggplants, use some as a side dish, then use and the rest as a part of the filling for fabulous pita sandwiches or as the base for a vegetarian entree.

Make double batches and freeze. You can save precious minutes at the end of a long work or school day if you take time on a weekend to make a soup or stew. Make a double batch and freeze in containers for future fast, healthy, delicious dinners.

Use leftovers to create new dishes. Don't throw leftovers away! Spruce up pasta or other whole grain bases with leftovers. Or, combine leftovers from several meals for a totally new dish!

Use timesaving equipment, such as slow cookers and pressure cookers. Simply start your slow cooker before you leave home in the morning, and you'll come home in the evening to a ready-cooked meal. Alternatively, a pressure cooker or Instant Pot can transform ingredients that usually take a long time to cook (like beans, rice and other whole grains) into table-ready dishes (soups, stews, risotto) in a fraction of the time.

Too busy to eat well?

EATING WELL is a major investment in your health and well-being. Consider this when you say "I don't have time to cook (or shop or meal plan)."

The good news is that when you implement some smart strategies, preparing nutritious, nourishing meals doesn't have to take a lot of time:

- **Learn how to cook** (if you don't know how already). Cooking is faster when you know what you're doing. If your skills are minimal, start by focusing on a few techniques you would like to learn, then make them your own. For example, making soups and stews, stir-frying, grilling, braising, roasting. Each of these are techniques that you can use to build a repertoire of go-to meals that you can cook confidently.

- **Organize your kitchen.** Ruthlessly get rid of things you don't need or use in your drawers, cupboards, pantry, refrigerator and freezer. (See the Kitchen Cleanout handout on the website)

- **Plan.** You may think it takes too much time to meal plan, but investing a bit of time upfront to sketch out a meal plan will save you time later in the week, because you can also shop more efficiently (preventing you from needing to run to the store and figure out what to feed yourself for dinner).

- **Shop online.** If taking your streamlined shopping list to the grocery store feels like too much, let your fingers do the shopping. More and more stores are offering online ordering and delivery.

- **Set aside a block of time.** Choose a three-hour block on the weekend where you can do some advance cooking and food prep for the week. You might feel raring to go on Friday evening, but more likely you'll end up choosing between morning, afternoon and evening on either Saturday or Sunday (see, you have seven time slots to chose from).

- **Use technology.** Slow-cookers can let the cooking happen unattended, while pressure cookers can cook grains, beans, soups, stews and most other things in the blink of an eye.

- **Use convenience foods wisely.** Frozen veggies, canned beans, rotisserie chickens, pre-washed salad greens can all make it easier to get a nutrition meal on the table, fast, without the added salt, sugar and fat that you'll find in takeout food and heat-and-eat meals.

- **Set firm mealtimes.** When you know when you'll be eating, it's easier to keep your cooking and other meal prep organized than when you are more loosey-goosey.

Chapter summary

When it comes to home cooking for better nutrition, there's truth to the adage "When you fail to plan, you plan to fail."

Here are the main takeaways from Chapter 11:

- Meal planning is a time investment that will save you time, stress and money many times over.
- Planning a perfect (for you) pantry can make grocery shopping and meal planning easier.
- With some thought and organization, you can get dinner on the table faster than you can pick up takeout. Home-cooked meals in minutes are possible!
- Let go of the idea that you're too busy to eat well. When there's a will, there's a way, with the help of some smart shortcuts.

Coming up in Chapter 12, Intuitive and Mindful Eating:

- Attuned eating
- Reclaiming intuitive eating
- Mindful eating: What are you hungry for?
- Mindless eating and digestion
- Getting started with mindful eating
- Identifying hunger
- Eating one raisin
- Normal eaters

PART 4

Where & How

"All great change in America begins at the dinner table."

— RONALD REAGAN

"When walking, walk. When eating, eat."

— ZEN PROVERB

CHAPTER 12

Intuitive and Mindful Eating

IF YOU WANT TO EAT in a way that nourishes your body with the food it needs to run really well, while enhancing your enjoyment of the food you eat, then intuitive and mindful eating are the paths to choose. Learning to eat intuitively and mindfully takes practice, and the more you've dieted in the past, the stranger it may feel to start to allow your own tastes, preferences and innate body wisdom guide your eating instead of external rules from diet culture.

In this chapter, I'll talk about:

- What **attuned eating** is, and how to tell if your eating needs a tune-up.
- The benefits of **reclaiming intuitive eating** instead of continuing to subscribe to external "rules" about how to eat.
- The basics of **mindful eating**, including the value of asking yourself what are you hungry for.
- Some simple tips for **getting started with mindful eating**.
- And some advice for **identifying hunger** if you've fallen out of touch with those natural cues.
- Some things you might not know about **mindless eating and digestion**.
- And finally, "**normal eaters,**" and why they are a rare and wonderful group that is worth joining.

Attuned eating

DO YOUR ATTUNED EATING SKILLS need a "tune up"? What is attuned eating, anyway? Attuned eating is similar (some people might say synonymous) with intuitive eating or mindful eating, which I'll talk about in more depth later in this chapter. Attuned eating isn't about external rules, it's about eating in the best way for your health and your life based on what you learn about yourself by tuning into:

- The way you feel when you eat (or don't eat) at certain times or intervals
- Why you eat, and how often it's for non-hunger reasons
  How you eat

Many people go through their days, weeks, months and years eating without a thought as to the when, why and how. Often the "what" is determined by external factors, such as dieting "rules" or whatever food happens to be close at hand. But the food you eat is too important to be an afterthought. When you put thought into what food nourishes both your body and your taste buds, it makes you feel good not just in the moment but after you eat and even further down the road

This is where food and mood journaling comes it. I'll be the first to admit that keeping a food journal isn't the most exiting of tasks. But I also know that food journaling is a tool worth pulling out of your toolbox when it makes sense. It's not about counting calories, it's about increasing awareness.

When you write down what you eat, when you eat it, your mood and whether there's anything notable going on around the time you are eating (extreme hunger, cravings, stress, eating while walking, eating while in the car, eating at a restaurant), you give yourself the ability to objectively look at your eating patterns.

- Are you going too long between meals (and getting too hungry)?
- Are you skipping breakfast and feeling tired mid-morning?
- Are you eating not because of hunger, but because you are bored, stressed or lonely?
- Are your food choices leaving you sleepy instead of energized?
- Are you often eating to the point of uncomfortable fullness?
- Are you in the habit of grabbing whatever food is handy, rather than making thoughtful food choices?

160

Reclaiming intuitive eating

WHAT DOES IT MEAN to eat intuitively? On a very basic level, it means eating for physical rather than emotional reasons most of the time (even intuitive eaters eat emotionally sometimes) and relying on your internal hunger and fullness cues rather than external cues to guide you, rather than relying on external cues like the time of day or the simple availability of food. It's a skill we were all born with, but most of us lost it at some point during childhood. It's a skill well worth relearning. On a deeper level, intuitive eating is an approach that:

- Teaches you how to create a healthy relationship with your food, mind, and body.
- Helps you become the expert of your own body by learning how to distinguish between physical and emotional feelings so you gain a sense of body wisdom.
- Guides you through the process of making peace with food and reducing "food worry" thoughts. It helps you know and accept that your health and your worth as a person don't change because you ate a food that you had labeled as "bad" or "fattening."
- Can open up a world of satisfying eating and a sense of food freedom.

The underlying premise of intuitive eating is that you will learn to respond to your inner body cues because you were born with all the wisdom you need for eating intuitively. On the surface, this may sound simplistic, but it is rather complex. Our inner wisdom is often clouded by years of dieting and food myths that abound in our culture.

For example, "Eat when you're hungry and stop when you're full" sounds like basic common sense, but if you have a history of chronic dieting or of following rigid rules about healthy eating, it can be quite difficult. To be able to return to your inborn intuitive eater, many of things need to be in place—most importantly, the ability to trust yourself!

Here is a summary of the 10 Principles of Intuitive Eating, from the book "Intuitive Eating" by Evelyn Tribole, MS, RD and Elyse Resch, MS, RD, FADA.

Reject the diet mentality. Throw out the diet books and magazine articles that offer you false hope of losing weight quickly, easily, and permanently. Get angry at the lies that have led you to feel as if you were a failure every time a new diet stopped working and you gained back all of the weight. If you allow even one small hope to linger that a new and better diet might be lurking around the corner, it will prevent you from being free to rediscover Intuitive Eating.

Honor your hunger. Keep your body biologically fed with adequate energy and carbohydrates. Otherwise you can trigger a primal drive to overeat. Once you reach the moment of excessive hunger, all intentions of moderate, conscious eating are fleeting and irrelevant. Learning to honor this first biological signal sets the stage for re-building trust with yourself and food.

Make peace with food. Call a truce, stop the food fight! Give yourself unconditional permission to eat. If you tell yourself that you can't or shouldn't have a particular food, it can lead to intense feelings of deprivation that build into uncontrollable cravings and, often, bingeing When you finally "give-in" to your forbidden food, eating will be experienced with such intensity, it usually results in Last Supper overeating, and overwhelming guilt.

Challenge the food police. Scream a loud "NO" to thoughts in your head that declare you're "good" for eating under 1000 calories or "bad" because you ate a piece of chocolate cake. The Food Police monitor the unreasonable rules that dieting has created. The police station is housed deep in your psyche, and its loud speaker shouts negative barbs, hopeless phrases, and guilt-provoking indictments. Chasing the Food Police away is a critical step in returning to intuitive eating.

Discover the satisfaction factor. The Japanese have the wisdom to promote pleasure as one of their goals of healthy living In our fury to be thin and healthy, we often overlook one of the most basic gifts of existence—the pleasure and satisfaction that can be found in the eating experience. When you eat what you really want, in an environment that is inviting and conducive, the pleasure you derive will be a powerful force in helping you feel satisfied and content. By providing this experience for yourself, you will find that it takes much less food to decide you've had "enough".

Honor your feelings without using food. Find ways to comfort, nurture, distract, and resolve your issues without using food. Anxiety, loneliness, boredom, anger are emotions we all experience throughout life. Each has its own trigger, and each has its own appeasement. Food won't fix any of these feelings. It may comfort for the short term, distract from the pain, or even numb you into a food hangover. But food won't solve the problem. If anything, eating for an emotional hunger will only make you feel worse in the long run. You'll ultimately have to deal with the source of the emotion, as well as the discomfort of overeating.

Respect your body. Accept your genetic blueprint. Just as a person with a shoe size of eight would not expect to realistically squeeze into a size six, it is equally as futile (and uncomfortable) to have the same expectation with body size. But mostly, respect your body, so you can feel better about who you are. It's hard to reject the diet mentality if you are unrealistic and overly critical about your body shape.

Exercise — feel the difference. Forget militant exercise. Just get active and feel the difference. Shift your focus to how it feels to move your body, rather than the calorie burning effect of exercise. If you focus on how you feel from working out (hopefully energized!), it can make the difference between rolling out of bed for a brisk morning walk or hitting the snooze alarm. If when you wake up, your only goal is to lose weight, it's usually not a motivating factor in that moment of time.

Honor your health with gentle nutrition. Make food choices that honor your health and taste buds while making you feel well. Remember that you don't have to eat a perfect diet to be healthy. You will not suddenly get a nutrient deficiency or gain weight from one snack, one meal, or one day of eating. It's what you eat consistently over time that matters— progress, not perfection, is what counts.

Potential pitfall

It's easy to turn intuitive and mindful eating into a diet if you treat the principles as all-or-nothing, pass-or-fail rules (for example, "I totally screwed up by eating when I wasn't hungry.") The process of tuning into to what, and how much, food your body and tastebuds need calls for gentle exploration and a sense of curiosity while leaving self-judgment at the door. (For example, "Hmmm…I just ate that granola bar and I wasn't even hungry. What's going on? Was my breakfast not satisfying tastewise? Was going to get a snack a way to delay tackling my overflowing inbox?") Be kind to yourself. You might think of learning to eat intuitively and mindfully like learning to play the piano: Some practice sessions might leave you thinking, "Hey, I sound OK!" while others leave you thinking, "I swear, I played like I have 10 thumbs!"

Mindful eating: what are you hungry for?

HOW OFTEN DO YOU pay attention to what you eat, while you're eating it? I mean, really pay attention. Do you often find that you finish the food on your plate without noticing or tasting, most of it? If your answer is "yes," you are not alone. The good news is that anyone can learn to eat mindful-ly…and the benefits are worth the effort!

What is mindful eating?

When you eat mindfully, you are aware and engaged in the present mo-ment, in a non-judgmental way. You are conscious of the act of eating. You slow down and savor each bite. You start eating because you are get-ting hungry. You stop eating when your body or taste buds tell you you've had enough. The Center for Mindful Eating (tcme.org) defines mindful eating as:

- Allowing yourself to become aware of the positive and nurturing opportunities that are available through food preparation and consumption by respecting your own inner wisdom.
- Choosing to eat food that is both pleasing to you and nourishing to your body by using all your senses to explore, savor and taste.
- Learning to be aware of physical hunger and satiety cues to guide your decision to begin eating and stop eating.
- Acknowledging responses to food (likes, neutral or dislikes) without judgment.

What is mindless (distracted) eating?

To eat mindlessly is to eat while you are distracted or lost in thought. You are operating on autopilot. You eat quickly and barely taste your food. You might start eating because you are hungry, but it might also be because you are bored, stressed, or just because you always eat lunch at 12:30. You stop eating when your food is gone.

Mindless eating is eating based on environmental cues, such as the presence of food, and eating triggers, such as stress. These cues and trig-gers can cause you to eat unhealthy foods, eat too much food, or both. Most people don't mindlessly eat carrot sticks. Minimizing mindless eat-ing cues can make it easier to tune into your body's true signals about what and how much to eat.

The benefits of mindful eating

Mindful eating is a skill that takes some practice, but the payoff can be great. Mindful eating can help you get back in touch with your body's signals of hunger, fullness and satisfaction. This makes it easier to put your fork down before you overindulge. Mindful eating can also help you enjoy your food more. When you make a point of tasting each bite, you get maximum pleasure from the experience of eating.

If you struggle with emotional, stress or comfort eating (which we'll cover more in Chapter 15), becoming more mindful can help you tune into your feelings and increase your self-awareness about whether what you really need is food…or something else. Over time, this can improve your ability to cope with uncomfortable feelings that lead you to food.

On a physical level, eating while distracted is similar to eating while you are feeling stressed (in other words, you body can't tell the difference between distraction and stress). This interferes with digestion, which means that your body can't make the most of the wonderful foods you are giving it! This can make you feel like you have less energy. Eating while distracted or stressed also contributes to increases in blood sugar levels, fat storage and chronic inflammation, while depressing your body's immune and detoxification systems.

Getting started with mindful eating

YOU DON'T HAVE TO PRACTICE mindfulness at every meal to benefit from it. You may find that it's easiest to start with select meals, such as those eaten alone. Here are some tips to help you start on a more mindful path:

Set a place at the table. Clear clutter off the kitchen or dining room table. Set out a plate, utensils and a napkin. If you can, use an attractive placemat or light a candle. This makes it easier to slow down and enjoy the act of eating.

Make your bites count. When faced with many food choices, ask yourself what you really want to eat. Take the time to choose food you really like and food that would satisfy you right now. Choose food that honors your taste buds and your body.

Sit quietly for a moment before picking up your fork. Take a few deep breaths and actually look at the food you are about to enjoy. What does it look like? Does it look appealing? Where does it come from? Is it a food you can recognize or is it a food-like substance (e.g. highly processed)? Briefly be aware of the sun, the rain and all of the other processes by which this food arrived in front of you today. Ask yourself if this is the food you really want. A brief pause to assess your food can give you lots of information about it.

If you usually eat quickly, practice slowing your pace. Slowing down while you are eating can help you truly taste your food so that you enjoy your food more fully. Slowing down also helps you be aware of when your hunger is becoming satisfied. Simple methods to help you slow down include putting down your fork or spoon between bites, pausing and taking a breath between bites, and chewing your food completely and swallowing before picking up your next bite (this also helps you digest the nutrients from your food).

Eat with all of your senses. Pay attention to the colors of the food. Notice the texture and sounds, the aroma and flavor. Is it crunchy, creamy, warm, cold, sweet, salty, spicy? Become fully present for the experience of eating and the pleasure that it can bring. Let all of your attention be on the complete range of sensations available in each bite and feel the joy. If you can't savor it, why eat it?

Pause halfway through your meal. Check in with how you feel. Is your belly full? Are you satisfied? Does the food still taste delicious? If you clean your plate and want more, wait five minutes, then decide if you are still hungry. You may discover you're no longer hungry even though there's food on your plate or you may discover you don't even like the food you're eating. Give yourself permission to stop—or to continue—based on what you discover.

Minimize multitasking while you eat. Eat at least some meals without distractions like the computer, television, handheld electronics, magazines, books or intense conversations. If you must eat with distractions, be aware of them, and make a point to bring your attention back to eating, tasting, and assessing your hunger and satiety several times throughout the meal.

Susan Albers, PsyD, author of several books
on mindful eating, suggests
the Four S's of Mindful Eating:

Sit down ("Only eat while off your feet")

Savor each bite (Smell, listen, look, touch, taste)

Slowly chew

Still your mind, stay in the moment, take a deep breath

Identifying hunger

INTUITIVE AND MINDFUL EATING are natural processes that often don't feel natural when you are first trying them out. You may find that you have trouble knowing for certain when you are hungry and when you are not hungry., especially if your days are chaotic, you have a long-standing habit of skipping meals, or you tend to eat in a grazing pattern (in effect "staying ahead" of your hunger). Any combination of the following may be experienced as hunger sensations or symptoms:

- Mild gurgling or gnawing in the stomach
- Growling noise
- Light-headedness
- Uncomfortable stomach pain
- Irritability
- Feeling faint
- Headache

When you "breath and belly check" before you eat, ask yourself:

- "Am I hungry?"
- "What's my hunger level?"
- "What am I hungry for?"

When you "investigate your hunger throughout your meal," ask yourself:

- "Has my body had enough?"
- "Am I eating just because there's more food?"
- "Can I stop before I get full?"

The feelings of hunger and satiety may be hard to identify at first. Keep checking and you will learn more about your body and what it needs and wants.

Hunger and Satisfaction Scale

1. Ravenous, almost painfully hungry (this is when you feel like you could eat the table top)
2. Very hungry!
3. Moderately hungry, feeling a physical sense of hunger (this is a good time to think about eating soonish)
4. Slightly hungry

5. Comfortable. Not physically hungry or full
6. Gently satisfied with the meal (mind and belly feel sated
7. Starting to get a feeling of fullness
8. A little too full, feeling like you could have stopped several bites ago
9. Way too full, "stuffed" to the point where it hurts

Mindless eating and digestion

DIGESTION IS A COMPLEX PROCESS that requires constant communication between your gut and your nervous system (especially the brain). That communication starts before we even start to eat, when we smell and see food and anticipate eating it. Once we start eating, it can take about 20 minutes before the brain receives the "I'm full" message from the stomach. Eating quickly and mindlessly can cause you to reach the point of fullness before you realize it, which can cause you to accidentally overeat.

Now I want to mention two terms that are often used interchangeably, although they shouldn't be: Satiation and satiety.

Satiation, or fullness, has to do with the weight or volume of food in your stomach. It's a physical experience. Satiety refers to the level of satisfaction you have after eating. It has to do with the visual, olfactory and even emotional experience of eating.

If you've ever noticed that some meals are rewarding and satisfying, even when they involve a relatively small amount of food, while other meals leave you feeling full but somehow hungry for more, that's satiety at work. This is one reason why many people eat past the point of satiation/fullness...they're not satisfied even with a full stomach.

When you are able to recognize the emotional experience of satiety before you recognize the physical experience of satiation/fullness, you generally remember the meal as being more pleasant and enjoyable. When the reverse happens, when fullness hits before satiety and you keep eating, this can lead to physical discomfort and feelings of "food guilt."

The practice of mindful eating helps shift the goal of eating to feeling satisfied rather than feeling full.

"Normal eaters"

WHEN YOU INVEST time and attention into cultivating your intuitive and mindful eating skills, you are also working on becoming a "normal" eater. I occasionally meet a normal eater—someone who has never had a single solitary eating issue. No restricting, no binging, no guilt, no "bad" and "good" foods. They eat nutritiously but also enjoy their food. This is uncommon today, sadly. So what does it look like to be a normal eater? This is how Ellyn Satter, developer of the Eating Competence model, defines normal eating:

Normal eating is going to the table hungry and eating until you are satisfied. It is being able to choose food you like and eat it and truly get enough of it—not just stop eating because you think you should.

Normal eating is being able to give some thought to your food selection so you get nutritious food, but not being so wary and restrictive that you miss out on enjoyable food.

Normal eating is giving yourself permission to eat sometimes because you are happy, sad or bored, or just because it feels good.

Normal eating is mostly three meals a day, or four or five, or it can be choosing to munch along the way. It is leaving some cookies on the plate because you know you can have some again tomorrow, or it is eating more now because they taste so wonderful.

Normal eating is overeating at times, feeling stuffed and uncomfortable. And it can be undereating at times and wishing you had more.

Normal eating is trusting your body to make up for your mistakes in eating. Normal eating takes up some of your time and attention, but keeps its place as only one important area of your life.

In short, normal eating is flexible. It varies in response to your hunger, your schedule, your proximity to food and your feelings.

— Ellyn Satter Institute: http://ellynsatterinstitute.org

Chapter summary

Being able to eat intuitively and mindfully can be incredibly freeing once you practice them enough to make the skills your own. It can take time, but then think about how much time it takes to obsess over diet rules? Here are the main takeaways from Chapter 12:

- Attuned eating is the best way to eat for your health, your life and your tastebuds
- Reclaiming intuitive eating is a return to an innate sense we had when we were very, very young.
- Mindful eating is a way of gently asking yourself what you are really hungry for.
- Getting started with mindful eating doesn't require eating with zero distractions at every meal!
- If you have trouble identifying hunger, be patient and keep listening to your body's cues. They're there, even if they're buried.
- Normal eating is not about being a perfect eater!

Coming up in Chapter 13, The Journey Ahead:

- Overcoming obstacles
- Preparing for setbacks
- Food pushers
- Dining out & socializing
- Staying on track

The Journey Ahead

HAVE YOU EVER THOUGHT, when the kids are back in school/when I'm not so busy at work/when I finally retire I'll start eating better and being more attentive to my health? The fact is that there's no perfect time to start taking care of your health and wellness needs. Life will always be busy or throw us curveballs, so learning how to anticipate possible obstacles and setbacks so they don't derail us, and learning how to get back on track as soon as possible when we are derailed (hey, it happens!), give you the flexibility to move towards better nutrition and health while still living your life.

In this chapter, I'll talk about:

- How to **overcome obstacles** that might get in the way of your efforts to form new habits, especially the **seven internal obstacles to success.**
- Why **preparing for setbacks** is smart, not fatalistic.
- How to deal with **food pushers** gracefully so you can respect your personal food boundaries.
- Why **dining out and socializing** doesn't mean that you can't eat for both nutrition *and* pleasure.
- Tips for **staying on track** towards your health and nutrition goals.

Overcoming obstacles

LIFE IS FULL OF BUMPS AND CURVES, even when you are at a place in your life that is "supposed to be" steady and calm. One of the real tricks to eating and living in a way that makes you feel good and supports your health, wellness and self-care goals is to make changes based on where you are right now, today, not to wait for an easier or more perfect tomorrow (more on perfection later in this chapter). To do that, you need to identify what obstacles are standing between you and change and then develop a strategy to overcome them.

Your obstacles may not be the same as the next person's, but there are some commonalities in the things that tend to trip us up.

Long work hours
This includes long commutes. When you are away from home for 12 (or more) hours a day, it can be awfully tempting to just pick up take-out for dinner and to skip yoga. Can you cook larger batches of food on the weekends for weekday leftover lunches/dinners? Can you designate some of those leftovers for nutritious home-cooked freezer meals? Can you find healthier takeout options? Can you exercise in the morning or at lunch?

Lack of kitchen confidence
As I talked about in Chapter 9, even basic cooking skills are well worth cultivating, as meals you make at home are almost always healthier than meals you get from restaurants or take-out joints. Can you take a cooking class? Can you get a cookbook with easy recipes and commit to mastering one at a time? Can you have a kitchen-savvy friend show you some basics? Remember, you don't have to be Julia Child to put a meal on the table.

History of physical inactivity
If you've never been consistently active, it can feel hard to reverse course, for many reasons. You may feel out of breath and lacking in stamina. You may have achy joints and weak muscles. You may feel uncoordinated and clueless about where to start. You may have avoided exercise all of these years because you frankly don't like it! Can you find a personal trainer who listens to you and takes into account your exercise history and any physical limitations? Can you find an friend to go on walks with so you don't feel alone? Do you need appropriate fitness shoes and clothes? Would you feel better exercising at home in private (there are many good DVDs and streaming videos for beginner exercisers)? Can you let go of any all-or-nothing ideas you might have and commit to starting out slow, even if it's for 5 minutes at a time?

Lack of support

There's no bones about it, it's harder to make healthy changes if you feel like you are going it alone. This is especially true if spouses/kids/room-mates aren't on board, but it's also hard if your coworkers and friends are plying you with cookies and suggesting going out for happy hour on a regular basis. Can you join a gym, sign up for a fitness class or take a cooking class so you're around others who are similarly interested in exploring wellness? Can you cultivate friendships with people who enjoy socializing while being active, instead of always needing food or alcohol to be involved?

Chronic health issues

If you are struggling with a health problem that limits your mobility or saps your energy, it makes it hard to prepare meals or be active. Can you go see a registered dietitian for one-on-one help? Can you ask your friends or family to help cook?

Lack of planning

I'm sure you've heard the saying, "When you fail to plan, you plan to fail." Well, it's totally true, especially when you are contending with busy schedules and end-of-work-day fatigue. Can you designate one weekday night to sketching out a plan for a week's worth of menus? Can you dedicate some time on the weekend (best not to leave this to Sunday evening) to grocery shop and then do some food prep and batch cooking? The time you invest in these activities will save you much more time (and probably money) during the rest of your week.

Seven internal obstacles to success

CULTIVATING HEALTHY LIFESTYLE HABITS like good nutrition and regular physical activity takes effort, especially if you have some deeply entrenched less-than-healthy habits. It's frustrating when you feel like you are putting in the effort but not seeing the payoff of improved well-being. Here are some pitfalls that can impede your progress toward better health:

Perfection

Perfection is the enemy of progress. Trying to eat perfectly or follow an ambitious fitness plan to the letter leads to all-or-nothing thinking: You're either perfect or you're a failure. This can lead to feelings of shame (see below). It can also block all progress while you search in vain for the perfect diet or exercise plan. Start small, start today, and keep moving forward.

Boredom

Eating the same foods prepared the same way day in and day out can become dull, even if you like those foods. There is comfort and convenience in sticking to a routine, especially when you are trying to cement new healthy behaviors into actual habits. However, once you feel like you're getting it down, expand your repertoire to keep things feeling fresh and interesting. Try a new recipe each week, or test out a fun exercise class or activity you've been curious about.

Aspirational thinking
Trying to go from a staple diet of restaurant, take-out and heat-and-eat foods to complicated home cooked gourmet recipes using fresh foods from the farmer's market is a lovely idea—that's likely to fail. Some people have the bandwidth to make broad, sweeping changes to their kitchens and their lives, but most make more progress by making simple, sustainable changes that will stick.

Insane thinking
By this, I mean doing the same thing you've always done and expecting different results. If you've lost weight in the past by cutting carbs, foregoing fat or standing on your head while eating, only to gain it all back—plus five pounds extra—in a year or two, why would you try it again and actually expect to keep the weight off this time?

Trying to control the wrong thing
You have direct control over whether you pack a nutritious brown bag lunch or make time for daily exercise. Taking actions like this each day will add up to larger health benefits, but you don't have direct control over the size or speed of your results. Tune into more subtle clues your efforts are working, such as sounder sleep, more energy or better digestion.

Succumbing to shame
Negative emotions like shame, disgust and self-directed anger are not effective motivators for change. When you don't like yourself, why should you take care of yourself? If a bad day or a bad week leads you to make choices that aren't in line with your nutrition and health goals, that doesn't mean you are weak or unworthy—it means you are human. See what you can learn from the experience, and move right on back to making choices that support your well-being.

Choosing superficial motivators
When you stop getting compliments about how healthy or fit you look, motivation can go out the window. Identifying and tapping into deeper sources of motivation, like having the energy to keep up with your kids (or grandkids) or staying fit so you can enjoy traveling, is more likely to

keep you on the path to continued progress.

Preparing for setbacks

SETBACKS ARE A LITTLE DIFFERENT from obstacles. Obstacles tend to be bigger and already present in your life. Setbacks tend to be less predictable and often are smaller (although huge setbacks can certainly happen…like breaking a leg!). Another key to success with making healthy changes that last is to learn how to roll with life's little ups and downs, and that includes preparing for inevitable setbacks. The key with setbacks is to:

Be aware that they can happen and likely will happen at some unforeseen time (unless you lead a particularly charmed life). Take that awareness, and resolve to not let setbacks completely derail you from your intentions. There's a big difference between two steps forward, one step back and two steps forward, "Oh, nuts, what just happened…oh, I might as well just forget about trying to be healthier." These are some setbacks that many people have to contend with at least occasionally:

Minor injury or illness

Yes, coming down with a cold or the flu or twisting your ankle puts a wrench in the works. Show yourself come compassion, nourish yourself teh best you can, and resume physical activity gently and gradually as soon as you are able. Don't be afraid to ask for/accept food prep and grocery shopping help from family and friends. You'll notice that I said minor injury or illness. If you suffer a major injury or illness, that becomes more of an obstacle than a mere setback, and will require a different set of strategies.

Vacations

Not only are you on unfamiliar turf and out of your usual routine, but odds are you are relying on restaurants more than you would at home. Add to that the somewhat celebratory atmosphere that usually accompanies a break from your usual workaday life, and it's easy to slide into a string of less-than-optimal food choices that leave you feeling less-than-your-best. I see vacations as a balancing act. On the one hand, traveling give you a chance to have new experiences, and food is part of that experience. On the other hand, when you want to feel good and stay energized, taking frequent or prolonged deviations from your food and activity routines can get in the way. Here are my top tips to have the best of both worlds when I travel:

- **Rent an apartment or condo.** This is more practical for vacations of several days or more than it is for quick trips, but this gives you an opportunity to not rely 100 percent on restaurants. You'll save money (both from the food and probably from lodging, as short-term rentals are usually less expensive than a hotel stay) and time, especially in the morning when you're eager to get out and sightsee (few things are easier than having a quick breakfast in your rental kitchen before you depart).

- **Eat vegetables and fruit.** Just because you are enjoying some foods that are more indulgent than what you would normally be eating doesn't mean you don't still benefit from the good stuff. Fruit and non-starchy vegetables are nutrient rich and water-rich, and can provide a refreshing balance to heavier fare.

- **Choose wisely.** Try the foods you've been looking forward to, but ignore those that you feel "meh" about. I've learned that I'm lukewarm about French macarons, so I can happily ignore those on my next trip to Paris.

- **Don't deprive yourself of food memories.** Are you really not going to have baguettes or pastries in Paris? No gelato in Italy? That would be sad, and you would likely regret it later.

- **Keep portions sizes reasonable, eat slowly and savor.**

- **Sightsee actively.** Don't rely on buses, trains and cars or taxis to deliver you from Point A to Point B (unless mobility is a real issue). Walking is often on of the best ways to sightsee. If I need to cover a very large distance, I might use transit to get me in the vicinity, but then I walk around all day (with park or café breaks as needed). Do I fret that my strength training and yoga routines go by the wayside when I travel? Not really, because I do so much walking. I know my muscles will get back in the game quickly once I'm home again.

Holidays

One reason most of us look forward to Thanksgiving and the holidays beyond is the food. Whether it's your mother's famous pumpkin pie or your uncle's stellar turkey dressing, food helps us celebrate and form lasting memories. But what happens if you want to have your pie and your mashed potatoes and not end up in a food coma?

- **Lighten…lightly.** Look for places to make tweaks that will go unnoticed. Can you reduce the amount of oil you use to sauté the onions? Can you replace some of the butter in the mashed potatoes with low-fat plain Greek yogurt or butter-milk for creaminess and flavor?

- **Add instead of subtract.** Bumping up the amount of veg-gies in the turkey dressing can lower calories while adding nutrients and preserving great taste. Balance out starch-heavy sides with a nice fall-winter salad (mixed greens, apples or pears, dried cranberries, pecans or walnuts, a sprinkle of blue cheese, vinaigrette) and extra vegetable dishes, such as roast-ed Brussels sprouts or green beans with almonds.
- **Streamline the menu.** Research shows that when offered more variety, most people eat more food. Keep the core favorites, add in more vegetables, then look for stragglers. I suggest ditching the dinner rolls, which are little more than a vehicle for butter. As far as starchy carbs go, the dressing and potatoes are much more delicious (at least I think so).
- **Bookend the meal.** It's nice to have something to nibble on while waiting for the feast, but traditional pre-meal offerings like cheese and crackers, bowls of nuts and hot hors d'oeuvres fill people up before the turkey hits the table. Instead, prepare the palate with a beautiful veggie tray with flavorful yogurt-based dips. Give the meal a strong finish by rethinking the number of desserts. Taking "just a sliver" of three different and equally tempting desserts usually adds up to a bigger portion than if there is just one wonderful offering.
- **Eat slowly.** It's ironic that we look forward to special hol-iday meals all year and spend hours (or days) preparing them, only to wolf down the fruits of that labor in minutes. When you don't give your first plate of food the attention it deserves, you don't fully taste it. That's likely to leave you wanting more, even if your stomach is full.
- **Don't drink your calories.** Eggnog, punch, soda, cider, wine, beer and cocktails all pack a calorie punch. Plus alco-hol can make us want to eat more. Try sparkling water with lemon or lime as a festive spacer—or substitute—beverage.
- **Frame the day.** Give holiday meals their due by eating nor-mally on the days surrounding it. Even holiday leftovers can be incorporated into a normal eating pattern...you don't have to actually reenact the big day! There's a difference between enjoying eating a little extra on a single day and allowing that excess to seep into several days—or weeks—of overdoing it.

Visiting family

Houseguests can also get in the way of your normal exercise schedule and put you in the path of indulgent foods that are not a part of your usual eating habits. This is where your new intuitive and mindful eating skills can come in handy. It also helps to try to fit in at least a little walking, and to make sure there are vegetables on the menu, even if you are expected to prepare particular family favorites that don't score high marks for nutrition

Unplanned work demands

You had dinner planned...but then you had to work late. You intended to get to the grocery store...but you've been working extra hours every day to get a big project done. How do you avoid relying on vending machines and greasy take-out?

- Keep some healthy snacks on hand (nuts, homemade trail mix) to tide you over and have a light meal when you get home (a salad, scrambled eggs with veggies).
- If you have to duck out of work for a take-out dinner, opt for more nutritious choices like salads (with protein), broth-based soups. Think protein and vegetables, with a moderate amount of carbohydrates (like beans or whole grains).
- If you tend to get slammed with a series of late nights on a regular basis, learn to lean more heavily on your pantry and freezer. You might find yourself using more frozen fruits and veggies than fresh, and that's OK.
- Investigate grocery delivery services. They may cost more than going to the store yourself, but they are almost certain to cost less than relying on take-out and restaurants.

Stress

During times of stress, it's harder to make nutritious food choices and take time to exercise. Your sleep may also suffer. If you have a tendency toward emotional eating, extra life stress can definitely cause setbacks, which may feel huge to you. Keep cultivating those tools in your stress-management toolbox. Deep breathing, meditation, visualization, laughter, and activities that bring you joy can help take the edge off stress and improve your health.

Food gifts

You make a point to create a nutritious home food environment, you bring your nutritious, delicious lunch to work...and then someone gives you a huge box of chocolates or brings a box of doughnuts into work. First of all, be mindful: Is this food something that you will really enjoy eating? If not, then pass it up (see the section on how to handle food pushers). If the gift is in your home, don't be afraid to give it away or throw it away… no one will know. Respect your personal boundaries for both health and taste preferences. If you eat food you don't want or need, it is going to waste. You are not a garbage disposal. (See food pushers below.)

Dinner disasters

Did that new recipe turn out so horribly that even the dog won't eat it? These things happen, and if you are a fledgling cook or are simply trying to bust out of your culinary comfort zone, they may happen more often. Have a plan for if they do. This is where a well-stocked pantry comes in handy.

Food pushers

FOOD CAN BE MANY THINGS. It can be nourishing, comforting, a source of pleasure or a celebration centerpiece. It can also be a catalyst for awkward feelings when someone tries to foist food on us that we're not hungry for or we simply don't want to eat. Although food pushers lurk year-round, food-centered holidays tend to encourage them. There's no reason to eat food you don't want. That's true even if you don't struggle to avoid holiday weight gain.

Food pushers come in two main categories: sharers and saboteurs. Some sharers use food as a way of expressing love and caring. Others may love to cook and enjoy showing off their skill by feeding others. Saboteurs tend to push food, particularly less-healthy food, onto those in their circle who they perceive as being thinner or healthier than they are.

With the Halloween-to-New Year's food gauntlet imminent, knowing how to deflect food pushers graciously is a skill worth cultivating. Sharers may view acceptance of their food offerings as validation of their feelings or their kitchen prowess, so tread lightly. Ditto for saboteurs, who might escalate their game in the face of rejection.

My primary strategy starts with a smile and a compliment. "Wow, that looks delicious." "Mmmm…is that cinnamon?" "Is this your famous chicken casserole?" Remember, most food pushers are trying to be nice. Next, deflect. "Too bad I'm not hungry right now." "Wow, I wish I hadn't just eaten lunch…I'm stuffed!" If you know they won't be watching you, you can say, "I'll have some in a little while." If they offer to wrap some up to send home with you, agree. You might really want it later, or you can just toss it. It's your call.

For repeat-offenders you know and love…like your grandma, develop a custom strategy. If Grandma spoons second helpings onto your plate without asking ("There's just a little left, finish it up."), take less food for your first helping and/or eat slowly. You can also try "Everything was so delicious! Boy am I full!" That gives you an excuse to not clean your plate twice. If you know dessert is always served immediately, with no time to digest, eat less of your entrée and go light on any appetizers (assuming you like the dessert being served).

Strategies that may backfire include telling pushers "Sorry, but I'm cutting back on sugar" or "My doctor says I need to watch how much salt I eat." They may feel like you're calling their food—or them—unhealthy. They may push even harder with lines like, "Come on, you have to enjoy yourself sometimes." As if that's your only chance to enjoy food—or life!

Also think twice before pretending to have a food allergy, because you run the risk of being caught out someday. ("I thought you said you were allergic to chocolate.")

It takes a little practice to say "no" to good food intentions, but stick with it. When you learn how to honor your needs while respecting the feelings of others, everyone wins.

Dining out and socializing

IT'S A COMMON SCENARIO…you feel like you have the nutrition thing figured out, you have your go-to nutritious meals and snacks, you keep your house stocked with the foods that make you feel energetic and well. And then you are faced with a restaurant meal or party, where you know that it will be harder to tune into hunger and fullness cues, and leave the party or restaurant feeling good, when portion sizes are large, or the hors d'oeuvres are plentiful. What to do?

First, I want to point out that how you approach dining out and socializing will likely be different if these are frequent occurrences vs. once-in-a while events. If life circumstance means that you must eat at restaurants frequently, then it's even more important to develop a strategy for making enjoyable food choices that also support your health and wellness goals. Here are some tips:

Pick the restaurant
This isn't always possible, especially if you dining out is part of your job (entertaining clients and whatnot) or if the meal is in honor of someone's birthday.

Don't deprive yourself
Some people decide to eat "really lightly" the day of a party or a big dinner out. This often translates to starving yourself. If you remember what I've

said in previous chapters about how allowing yourself to become ravenous makes it harder to make good food choices, then you'll understand
while compensating for high-calorie party food by trying to exist on air
and water at breakfast and lunch is not the best idea. Continue to eat
when you are hungry and aim to stop eating when you are satisfied. If you
do any compensation, you might simply make your day's food choices
extra-nutritious (lots of veggies, etc.) to provide some balance, but please
don't go hungry!

Eat intuitively
Just because you aren't eating at home doesn't mean that you can't eat
in response to hunger and satisfaction cues. Just because you're served a
huge portion doesn't mean you have to eat it all if it's going to leave you
feeling uncomfortably full. If it makes sense to take it home for leftovers,
then hooray, you have a tasty lunch to look forward to. But it's OK to leave
food behind, too. Be mindful of the "I paid for it, so I need to eat it" trap,
or the "Clean Plate Club" trap. Eating food you don't need and possibly
don't even enjoy helps no one.

Eat mindfully
Eating mindfully is always a good thing, but that's even truer when you
are eating food that you might consider a "treat." Being mindful will help
you get maximum enjoyment as well as making it easier to know when
you've had enough.

Include vegetables
Just like I mentioned when I was talking about vacations in the "Preparing for Setbacks" section, just because you are eating foods that are more
indulgent than your normal choices doesn't mean you shouldn't fit in the
nutritious stuff.

Order what you really want
If a few choices are equally appealing, go with the more nutritious choice.
If a few choices are equally appealing, but one choice will make better
leftovers, then go with that choice.

Don't be a sheep
Just because everyone else is ordering an appetizer and dessert, doesn't
mean that you have to, too. You know the entrée will be more than enough
food. However, if your party is game for sharing an appetizer and dessert,
that's a great way to try a dish without ending up feeling overfull.

Split a meal
Even if the restaurant charges a plate fee for sharing, it's worth it.

Watch the alcohol
Imbibing with abandon makes it easier to overeat, not to mention the fact that alcohol is not calorie-free!

Don't let your eyes be bigger than your stomach
I can't tell you how many times my husband and I have been out for dinner and he wants to order this, and this, oh…and that and that. My response is always the same, "Dude, we only have one stomach each!" I'm always right…and he admits it! When we go his way, we either end up too full or end up wasting a lot of food (this scenario often happens when we're traveling and can't take the leftovers with us).

Go back to business as usual
Even if you end up indulging heavily at that meal or party (whether intentionally or accidentally), tomorrow is a new day, and your next meal is a new meal. Don't start playing the blame-shame-guilt game. If you planned to keep it moderate, but you didn't, adopt an attitude of curiosity and ask yourself what happened. This may help you make choices that feel better on the next go-round. In any case, if you consider the event a setback, don't let it derail you. Just keep moving forward.

Staying on track

IF THE ROAD TO SUCCESS is paved with good intentions, I'll wager that a good 75 percent of that pavement is poured from the intent to eat "right," move more and improve health. While people don't set out to purposefully sabotage their efforts, an awful lot of derailment goes on, nonetheless. Sometimes it's because we're just not thinking…sometimes it's because we're overthinking. I've made every one of the following mistakes at some point. What about you?

Failing to plan
Rome wasn't built in a day, and those sketchy eating habits you'd like to change weren't either. Changing habits can be hard work, so thinking you can turn yourself into a healthier, more balanced eater without a game plan is guaranteed to leave you spinning your wheels. If you don't have a plan, you will slip into "default mode" (aka your old habits) time and time again. "I want to eat healthier" is vague. "I will bring fresh fruit to work for snacks instead of hitting the vending machine" is a plan.

Not having a nutritional gatekeeper
Most of us tend to eat more of what is close at hand, so if chips, sugary beverages and pints of ice cream are always in the house, guess what's

probably going down the hatch. While skilled intuitive eaters can pretty much have any food in the house and take it or leave it, if you're not quite there yet, it can be helpful to keep trigger foods out of the house. That doesn't mean those foods are off limits...just that you don't have them at your fingertips. Stock your pantry and kitchen with nourishing foods that taste good and keep you feeling good. This is especially important if you find you often arrive home from work ravenous, or if you are prone to eating out of stress or boredom.

Being a human garbage disposal

Classic examples are nibbling left-behind food off your kids' plates when cleaning up and letting your grandmother serve you that "that last little bit" so it doesn't go to waste...even though you're full. Do you ever eat crackers that have gone stale or day-old break room doughnuts? Do you eat enough to get your "money's worth" at buffet brunches? Please stop. Being a member of the Clean Plate Club rarely does anyone any favors.

Not seeing the forest for the trees

Do you fuss about eating the latest, greatest exotic "superfood"? Try focusing your efforts—and food dollars—on including ample amounts of familiar vegetables and fruits into your meals and snacks each day. If you find yourself putting off eating more nutritiously while you fret about what ratio of carbs/protein/fat you "should" eat, shift gears and regain dietary sanity by getting down to business with the basics: Eating more vegetables, cutting back on junk food and learning to eat intuitively.

Making every day "special"

There are a handful of days of the year that warrant a little food splurging. Your birthday. Your anniversary. Major holidays. A rare visit from dear, long-distance friends. You get the idea. You'll notice I didn't mention "Fridays" or "crazy work days." Balanced eating leaves room to enjoy cake on your birthday and your family's secret-recipe stuffing on Thanksgiving. But if you celebrate every coworker's birthday and minor holiday with rich desserts and calorific meals, you probably won't feel as well as you would like.

There's more to nourishing yourself well than this, of course, but seeing these traps and learning to sidestep them can greatly improve the quality and quantity of what you put in your mouth. And that can lead to better health.

Chapter summary

I hope this chapter reminds you that it's about progress, not perfection. Making positive changes for your nutrition and health, and maintaining those changes over time, is much easier if you allow yourself some bad days (or weeks) and missteps but keep your eye on the big picture of what you want for yourself.

Here are some of the main takeaways from Chapter 13:

- Overcoming obstacles is mostly about mindset.
- No one leads a charmed life, so preparing for setbacks will help you stay true to your goals.
- It really is possible to deal with food pushers gracefully and respect your food boundaries.
- Dining out and socializing does not have to be scary or a straight shot to overindulgence.
- Staying on track isn't about never getting off track, it's about course correcting as soon as possible.

Coming up in Chapter 14, Being A Savvy Nutrition Consumer:

- Who can you trust?
- Nutrition in the news
- Be immune to health halos

Being A Savvy Nutrition Consumer

ONE OF THE BENEFITS of learning to tune into—and trust—your body and your tastebuds is that you become relatively immune to the confusing nutrition news out there. There are a lot of voices in the nutrition sphere—some worth listening to, and some not—and boy, those voices can be loud! I have a Master's degree in nutrition, but even I feel confusion from time to time (a deep dive into the research literature usually cures that). I hope to help you become more empowered so you can make informed decisions and not be swayed by food and nutrition trends.

In this chapter, I'll talk about:

- Some solid advice to decide **who you can trust** (besides yourself) for nutrition information.
- How to not get whiplash when reading about **nutrition in the news,** with specific tips to keep in mind when reading about nutrition research.
- Why it's a good thing to be **immune to health halos,** since a lot of foods that have halos aren't all they are cracked up to be.

Who can you trust?

THE VERY FACT THAT you are reading these words right now means that you are interested in nutrition and health, and it's a pretty good bet that my words aren't the only words on the topic that you have read, or will read. It's no secret that there's a lot of nutrition information out there, more now than ever thanks to the internet. The good news is that reliable nutrition information is right at your fingertips. The bad news is that it's harder to separate the wheat from the chaff.

Everybody eats, so everybody has an opinion about food and nutrition. While I think each one of us can become the ultimate expert on our own nutrition (especially as we cultivate intuitive and mindful eating skills), many people take it upon themselves to act as some sort of nutrition expert for whoever's listening. So, who has the "right" to provide nutrition advice? It's a complicated issue, both in terms of the who and the what. As for "who," at the top of the heap, we have:

- Registered dietitian (RD) and registered dietitian nutritionist (RDN). Credentialed by the Commission on Dietetic Registration of the Academy of Nutrition and Dietetics (AND).
- Certified nutrition specialist (CNS). Certified by the Certification Board for Nutrition Specialists (CBNS).

The academic curriculum for both RDs/RDNs and CNSs is science-based and rigorous, and individuals with those credentials complete at least 1,000 hours of supervised practice experience and pass a multi-hour exam. To maintain these credentials, individuals must keep up with continuing education. They are the only nutrition professionals who can legally provide medical nutrition therapy (MNT). RDs/RDNs must have at least a bachelor's degree in nutrition from an accredited university (this will be changing soon to a minimum of a master's degree). CNSs must have at least a master's degree, but there is some concern about how closely the CBNS screens applicants to assure that their degree came from an accredited university.

Further down, we have everyone from personal trainers to yoga teachers to health coaches to acupuncturists to health food store employees to supplement store salespeople to chefs to bloggers to your next-door neighbor (not necessarily in that order). Here are a few "nutrition credentials" you may have heard of:

- **Holistic Nutritionist.** Has a degree from an approved holistic nutrition program and 500 hours of professional experience. They do not practice medical nutrition therapy. Certified by the Holistic Nutrition Credentialing Board, a division of the National Association of Nutrition Professionals.

- **Certified Health Coach.** This is the certification given out by the Institute of Integrative Nutrition, a year-long online course that has been a little controversial, to say the least (they've been accused of teaching students more about marketing themselves than they actually teach about nutrition). One good description I've seen of health coaches, generally (because there are other online programs that offer health coach certifications), is that a health coach is to a dietitian nutritionist as a life coach is to a psychologist.
- **Certified Clinical Nutritionist (CCN).** This sounds good, but this certification offered by the Clinical Nutrition Certification Board promotes some quite dubious health practices, and online training rather than real-world experience.
- **Certified nutritionist (CN).** This one can be confusing, because some states (including Washington state) allow individuals who have an advanced degree in nutrition, but who did not go through the additional training to become a registered dietitian, to be certified nutritionists (CNs). However, CN can also mean that the individual has completed a 6-course distance-learning program offered through American Health Science University and passed a proctored exam. This particular CN certification has close ties to the health food industry.
- **Certified nutrition consultant (CNC).** The only requirement to become a CNC is to have a high school diploma or GED and pass a series of 11 open-book tests. The credential comes from the American Association of Nutrition Consultants, which sounds all nice and official, but this credential is pretty much bogus.

Unfortunately, the term "nutritionist" is pretty much meaningless, because almost anyone who's taken a few online classes can call themselves one! The bottom like is that dietitians can call themselves nutritionists, but nutritionists cannot call themselves dietitians.

So that covers the "who," and now for the "what": Few people would quibble if your personal trainer/favorite blogger/next-door neighbor touts the benefits of eating more vegetables, but beyond the most general and universal (read: common sense) nutrition advice, it becomes stickier.

Not all dietary plans are appropriate for all people. That can be true for people with no existing health problems, but it's especially true for people who have a chronic disease or other serious health problem. When you are dealing with using nutrition to treat disease, that falls under medical nutrition therapy. That is not something to take lightly.

A special mention about doctors

It's an unfortunate fact that there is very, very little nutrition curriculum in medical school. What little there is tends to be in the context of how carbohydrates affect blood sugar or fats affect blood cholesterol (this is what I've been told by more than a few doctors). Some doctors have taken it upon themselves to learn more about nutrition because they realize that food can be good medicine and see the benefit of using diet to aid treatment when possible (instead of automatically picking up the prescription pad), but this is the exception, sadly. In my experience, many doctors fall prey to the same thinking as many non-doctors: If eating this or not eating that works for me, it must work for everyone. I've known doctors who tell all their patients to avoid gluten, even though this recommendation is NOT supported by science!

Nutrition in the news

PRETTY MUCH EVERY DAY, there are headlines about research studies involving nutrition and health, or articles about food and nutrition trends. When these appear in legitimate print or online publications, it's easy to take them as gospel and start wondering if you should change your personal habits accordingly. Maybe you do decide you should start eating less fat, less meat, less carbs, fewer eggs, or whatever the study results suggest—only to read a month later that a different study suggests the opposite!

If you dig in to the scientific literature on the role of diet in preventing disease and promoting overall good health, it can be frustrating at times. While lab (petri dish and test tube) and animal testing tell us a lot about how certain foods or even specific compounds in foods (for example, phytonutrients in plant foods) can help us stay healthy, when you look at research using actual living, breathing humans, the results can be all over the map. Why is that? One reason is that human studies that look at diet and disease use free-living humans! There are two main types of research studies;

Epidemiological studies survey subjects periodically about what they eat using some sort of a dietary assessment tool, and then they watch and wait to see who develops disease and who doesn't, and determine if there are common dietary patterns between the subjects who stay healthy and the subjects who don't. Trouble is, things other than nutrition affect health. Randomized control trials tell one group of people (the experimental group) to eat a certain way, and another group (the control group) to just keep on eating their usual diet. Which group a subject is assigned to is random. It also may not be possible to have people stick to their assigned diet for long enough to really get good answers, because diseases like diabetes, heart disease and cancer can take years or decades to develop.

Humans are not lab rats

It isn't possible to get a 100 percent accurate picture with either type of study. People may not remember exactly what they ate. They may fudge a bit so it looks like they eat better than they really do. The experimental subjects may not adhere to their plan. The control subjects may improve their diets (even though they were told not to) because they are aware they are being studied.

Basically, unless you keep your human subjects locked in a lab and totally control everything they eat (and how much they sleep, exercise, stress out, smoke, drink alcohol, etc.), there is an element of chance in even the most carefully designed study.

Another factor to consider is what type of humans were used in the study. In other words, if the study used healthy males in their 20s, the results may not apply very well to women in their 50s who have already started to develop some health problems (such as elevated blood sugar, blood pressure or blood cholesterol). In general, the larger and more diverse (age, gender, health status, ethnicity) the group being studied, the more likely that the results are meaningful for the rest of us.

The role of genes

And then there's our genes. While our genetic predisposition to cancer or other diseases isn't necessarily our destiny (that's where diet and lifestyle can tip the scales), it does play a role. People who have no genetic predisposition to cancer and live a healthy lifestyle are going to be less likely to develop cancer than people who do have that predisposition but live a healthy lifestyle.

Also, our genes may affect how much benefit we get from powerhouse foods like broccoli and berries. Our genes contain the codes for building specific proteins, and some of those proteins (enzymes are one example) are responsible for making use of the various elements of the food we eat. That means you may benefit more from broccoli than your neighbor, or vice versa.

The gut microbiota

Another reason is our gut microbiota. There are certain parts of our food (especially plant foods) that our bodies don't digest by themselves. That's the job of the bacteria that live in our intestine. There are certain types of fiber, for example, that don't benefit us directly. Rather, it's the byproduct of digestion by our friendly bacteria that is beneficial to health.

The composition of our microbiota varies depending on many factors, including diet, medication use, stress, and so on. I know of research going on right here in Seattle that is looking at how people metabolize flax seeds. It may turn out that some people benefit from putting flax on their oatmeal and in their smoothies, while others don't. Wouldn't it be nice to know which camp you fall into? I don't know anyone who actually enjoys flax…it's just kind of neutral.

The big picture

All of this uncertainty and individual diversity partially explains why we are encouraged to eat a variety of vegetables, fruits, whole grains, beans and other healthy foods. Eating a varied diet ensures that our bodies get the full spectrum of vitamins, minerals, fiber and phytonutrients. While this is important generally, it may also be directly important if it turns out that you personally benefit from broccoli but not berries, and you'd been avoiding broccoli but eating berries every day.

The field of nutrigenomics (how our genes interact with the foods we eat) is very exciting, and still very new. The hope is that continued research will make personalized nutrition more than just a dream, and that we will be able to truly eat for our genes if we choose to. Until then, I'm hedging my bets by eating mostly plants, and a wide variety of them.

Nutrition science: more tortoise than hare

Whenever you read about findings from a nutrition or health research study, keep in mind that science rarely (if ever) comes up with findings that present a true paradigm shift in what was previously thought to be true. Often, if a single study has radically different findings than what previous studies on the topic have found, there's something wrong with that study!

That said, science is ever-changing, as researchers find answers to some questions, prompting them to ask new or more detailed questions. In general, science evolves slowly, and it's more important to consider the entire body of research on a certain topic, rather than the results of one specific study. For example, there is a huge body of research on traditional Mediterranean-style diets, which as a whole show benefits for preventing and reducing heart disease, type 2 diabetes, weight gain and so on. However, within that body of research are some individual studies that, for whatever reason, did not find a connection between that type of diet and positive health outcomes.

Be immune to health halos

WHAT IS A "HEALTH HALO"? It's a phenomenon in which there is a halo effect on certain foods or brands, causing them to be perceived as healthy, even if they aren't. Health halos frequently lead to eating too much of a particular food because of false assumptions that it's healthier or has fewer calories than it really does.

How do foods and brands develop a health halo? Marketing. One reason is that these foods tend to come packaged with health claims and other marketing messages. When you're trying to make healthful choices in a hurry, these messages can fool you into thinking you've hit a nutritional home run.

Research shows that when someone thinks a food is healthy (due to words or images on the label or other marketing materials or for other reason) they tend to eat more of it. Words like "low-fat," "low-carb," "sugar-free," "no added sugar," "no trans-fats," "no high-fructose corn syrup," "gluten-free" and "natural" often have that affect.

Similarly, if a food has achieved popularity as a superfood, then the health halo will follow it even if it's used as an ingredient in an otherwise processed, not-so-healthy food (kale, coconut and acai berries are a few that come to mind). Here are five more "healthy-sounding" foods to be aware of:

- **Multi-grain.** This doesn't mean what you think it means. Multi-grain means is that the bread, cracker or other product is made from more than one type of grain. It doesn't mean that those grains are whole grains. Sadly, each grain in a multi-grain product may be refined, stripped of its fiber and nutrients. What you want to see is the word "whole" in the list of ingredients on the Nutrition Facts panel. "Whole wheat flour" or "whole grain flour" means the fiber and nutrients are intact. "Wheat flour," "rye flour" and the like means they are gone, baby, gone.
- **Yogurt.** Do you think cellophane-wrapped snack cakes are a health food? Well, some yogurts have more sugar than those eternally shelf-stable marvels. Yogurt can be a very healthful food, but it can also be nutritionally comparable to dessert—which might not be what you want when it's time for breakfast or a healthy snack. Read labels to find variet-

ies that are lower in sugar, or add a dab of jam or squirt of honey to plain yogurt. In a pinch, cut the sugar by simply leaving most of the "fruit at the bottom" behind!

- **Salads.** Forget the name—the "devil" is in the ingredients. Add too much creamy dressing, cheese, nuts, dried fruit and croutons and you can quickly bury the poor salad greens while serving yourself more food than your body needs. The worst offenders are many of the massive main-dish salads served in chain restaurants. Build a smarter salad by loading up on veggies and using modest amounts a few favorite higher-calorie extras.

- **Energy bars and drinks.** These products claim to "fuel your workout," but many of them are nutritionally equivalent to a candy bar or sugary cola. If you appreciate the portability of bars when you're on-the-go, read the Nutrition Facts box and the list of ingredients. Look for the bars that have the shortest ingredient list and the most natural, "real food" ingredients. There are a few brands that contain little more than a delicious mix of ground up dried fruits, nuts and seeds.

- **Smoothies.** These meals-in-a-glass can be 1,000-calorie sugar bombs with the wrong ingredients. Say yes to real fruits (and even vegetables) and low-fat or nonfat milk or yogurt (or dairy alternatives). Say no to sugar-laden fruit juices, ice cream, whole milk or yogurt and added sugars like chocolate syrup.

Don't forget that businesses can have health halos, too. Whole Foods bills itself as "America's Healthiest Grocery Store," but they sell a lot of heavily processed foods (potato chips, ice cream, fried foods in the hot bar) that don't contribute to nutrition. Similarly, Subway has the reputation as being a healthy fast-food option, but studies show that when people feel virtuous by going to Subway instead of, say, McDonalds, they are more likely to feel justified in splurging on chips, soda and cookies to go with their sandwich. That's not so intuitive!

Chapter summary

Nutrition can be as confusing—or as clear and simple—as you want it to be. One excellent way to cut the confusion factor is to learn what messages you can just tune out.

Here are the main takeaways from Chapter 14:

- With so many alleged "nutrition experts," it's important to know who you can trust.
- Most nutrition news is not worth changing your habits over.
- When you stop looking for magic bullets, you become immune to health halos

Coming up in Chapter 15, Head Games:

- Stress and emotional eating
- Coping with cravings
- Food addiction
- Disordered eating

PART 5

Why

"The spirit cannot endure the body
when overfed, but, if underfed,
the body cannot endure the spirit."

– ST FRANCES DE SALES

Head Games

ALTHOUGH OUR PRIMARY reason for eating is to fuel our bodies, with pleasing our tastebuds running somewhere in second place, in fact there are a lot of reasons why we eat. Stress. Cravings. Emotions. Boredom. Impulse (I see food therefore I eat it). While eating for reasons other than sustenance and joy isn't a big deal if it doesn't happen very often, if it's a frequent driver of your eating behavior it may contribute to overeating and get in the way of finding more meaningful ways to soothe or entertain yourself.

In this chapter, I'll talk about:

- **Stress and emotional eating** are parts of life, but you can cultivate tools to reduce their grip on you.
- How to get better at **coping with cravings**, and how to figure out if it's a true craving...or a mere impulse.
- More tips on **finding and feeling hunger**, especially when it's all tangled up in your cravings.
- Why the notion of **food addiction** is controversial, and may sometimes be a self-fulfilling prophecy.
- How to tell the difference between **disordered eating** and an eating disorder.

197

Stress and emotional eating

DO YOU SOMETIMES eat to soothe or comfort yourself when you're under stress or when you're feeling sad, anxious, overwhelmed, bored or lonely? Do you feel like you have a pretty good handle on how to eat nutritiously, yet find yourself frequently snacking on cookies? If so, you are far from alone. The reason that so many people engage in these and other forms emotional eating is that it works…sort of.

The rush of sugar from candy or cupcakes, the crunch of salty potato chips, the creaminess of ice cream or macaroni and cheese, each of these can make you feel better in the moment, whether because they remind you of happier times or because they serve as a distraction from what's bothering you. In that way, emotional eating works as a short-term solution. What emotional eating doesn't do is get to the heart of what's eating you. It doesn't get to the source of your stress or sadness. It doesn't offer you a long-term solution.

Is emotional eating to blame for weight gain?

It's a truth universally acknowledged that emotional eating contributes to weight gain—but is this a false truth? Many patients come to my office with the "emotional eater" label firmly affixed to themselves, convinced that if they could solve that problem, all their food and weight woes would evaporate. That's rarely the case—because emotional eating isn't about the food.

The concept of emotional eating was born in the 1960s, the original idea being that emotional eaters couldn't tell the difference between hunger and the physical sensations that accompany unpleasant emotions. Today, we often think of emotional eating as "feeding our feelings." But even though we think emotions drive us to overeat, research suggests that may be more perception than reality.

Believe it, then become it? There are a number of emotional eating self-assessment scales that quiz you about how often you feel the urge to eat in response to emotions. The problem with self-assessment is that it's hard to accurately recall past emotions, past eating behavior, and whether there was a connection between the two. Your score may reveal more about how you think your eating is tied to your emotions than your actual eating behavior.

Calling yourself an emotional eater could reflect conflicted feelings about your food choices—whether the amount or the perceived healthfulness—even if your eating habits aren't all that different from someone who doesn't identify as an emotional eater. Research suggests that people who are concerned about their eating behavior may retrospectively attribute overeating to emotions or stress, because emotional eating has become a commonly accepted explanation for food choices we judge as less-than-desirable.

As for those emotional eaters who actually overeat, they are also more likely to overeat when experiencing other food cues, including simply being around food. Research does show that emotional eating is associated with higher body weights and more weight gain—but it's also associated with dieting. And that's no coincidence.

A response to restriction? Dieting, or any restriction of amount or type of food, can lead to emotional eating due to physical and psychological deprivation. Indeed, research shows that former and current dieters are more likely to describe themselves as emotional eaters, while those who have never dieted tend to avoid food when experiencing stress or strong emotions due to the appetite-squelching fight-or-flight response.

Physical deprivation is when you don't eat enough and you're biologically hungry. This may make you feel like you shouldn't be feeling hungry because they ate enough food according to whatever food or dieting rules you're following, making it easy to blame yourself and label the eating you're doing as "emotional" instead of blaming the diet for making you so physically deprived that you can't help but eat.

Psychological deprivation can happen when you've placed a certain food is off-limits, making it "forbidden." When you eat that food, you may still feel deprived even after you're physically full and satisfied, so you keep eating that food and end up feeling overly full—and then label the experience as "emotional eating." The truth is that making the food forbidden in the first place caused the eating.

In a chicken-or-egg scenario, food restriction makes people more likely to overeat in response to emotional cues, but emotional eating can cause distress and guilt, potentially leading to dieting in an attempt for control. What comes first? That's difficult to say. Further muddying the waters is the fact that weight gain can cause feelings of failure, which may lead to the desire to soothe yourself with food.

Is emotional eating always a problem? There's no denying that emotional eating does offer temporary relief from uncomfortable feelings, or no one would do it, and eating in response to emotions is completely normal some of the time. However, if you are distressed about your relationship with food in general—maybe because you are caught in a restrict-binge cycle from putting certain foods off-limits and then eating, or over-eating, them—then seeking help may be worthwhile. That's especially true if you're bingeing regularly in a way that's hindering your life and causing you pain.

Of course, psychological deprivation doesn't just stem from food restriction—it can come from restriction in other areas of your life, like sleep, social connection, self-care or simple down time. This may sound odd, but some experts call emotional eating a gift, a clear signal that your needs aren't being met, that something needs to change. Consider it the canary in the coalmine.

Awareness of when you are eating to self-soothe is a first step to breaking unhelpful eating patterns, but curiosity is also key. If you consider yourself an emotional eater, it's worth asking yourself what role dieting and deprivation might be playing. If you recognize that you do restrict yourself from eating certain things and you feel deprived, consider that the deprivation might actually be at the root of what you think of as emotional eating—not emotions at all. Here are a few techniques, that may help ease the effects of emotional eating:

- **Label your feelings.** The very act of identifying the emotion you're experiencing can help release it's hold on you.
- **Ask yourself what you really need.** Do you really need a cookie, or do you need to calm yourself.
- **Imagine the aftermath.** Visualize eating to soothe yourself. How long do the good feelings really last? Research has found that eating comfort foods may not improve mood any faster than eating nothing at all.
- **Open your toolbox.** What other hobbies or activities can you engage in to help you feel better?

Why emotional eating?

So how do we end up as emotional eaters, anyway? If you think it's because you don't have willpower, think again (willpower is very unreliable, in any case). It certainly doesn't help that fast, cheap, non-nutritious food is available practically everywhere—there's a fast-food restaurant on almost every corner, and even office supply stores sell candy bars.

Many of us are short on time and short on effective coping skills, and food can provide a much-needed break at the end of a busy day. When you were a child, if your parents or other caretakers used food to make you feel better (like a cookie when you skinned your knee) or as a reward (like cake every time you got a good grade), then these patterns are likely to follow you into adulthood…especially if you didn't get a lot of hugs or non-food sources of validation.

Feelings of deprivation can make you more likely to eat for emotional reasons. This includes allowing yourself to become overly hungry by skipping meals or undereating at meals (as is often the case when dieting). This is where practicing intuitive and mindful eating can help. When you eat intuitively, you honor your hunger. When you eat mindfully, you actually notice your food as you are eating it, which increases satisfaction and makes you less likely to head back to the kitchen to try to satisfy unmet (food) needs.

Coping with cravings

FOOD CRAVINGS ARE A FUNNY THING. Some people think that cravings means their bodies need nutrients found in the food they're fixating on ("I'm craving chocolate. I must be low in...zinc.") Other people see cravings as a sign of weakness, and either try to white knuckle it, or throw up their hands and declare themselves powerless. While cravings could be based on a nutritional need, most stem from other factors. So should you indulge cravings...or ignore them? The answer depends on what your craving is really telling you.

Cravings vs. impulses

Some cravings would be better described as an urge or impulse. A true craving is more of a slow burn—like when you have a yen for a favorite dish or cuisine that you haven't enjoyed for a while—that will smolder until you eventually satisfy it. An impulse is more of a flash in the pan—it comes on suddenly and will burn out on its own if you let it.

Unfortunately, our brains seem to be more wired to respond to impulses than to think beyond them. One technique for dealing with impulse-type cravings is to "surf the urge." To do this, imagine your craving as an ocean wave. Watch it as it builds gradually, getting stronger and stronger until it peaks (or crests) then gradually dissipates. Rather than deny the urge, actively surf it. Having the experience of watching the urge fade can make it easier to handle impulsive cravings when they next arise.

If your craving for, say a cookie just won't go away, get the best cookie you can find, and sit and savor it. What doesn't work is chasing the craving with foods you consider more "acceptable." If what you truly want is a cookie, all the apples or cinnamon rice cakes in the world won't satisfy it.

Environmental cues

Do you crave popcorn the moment you step into a movie theater? Grab a snack every time you lounge in front of the television? Get the urge for a cookie each day at 3 p.m.? If you've come to associate certain times, places or activities with a particular food, what likely started as a craving has morphed into mindless eating then on to pure habit. To untangle yourself from this Pavlovian response to food, practice asking yourself "Am I hungry?" whenever you have the urge to eat. If the answer is "no," ask yourself, "Why do I want to eat this?" If your answer is something like, "Because it's there" or "Because its what I always do," consider experimenting with not having the food to see how it feels.

Emotional or psychological needs

Do you crave ice cream or pasta when you're feeling stressed, sad, angry or lonely? A 2014 study co-authored by psychologist Traci Mann, author of "Secrets of the Eating Lab," found that eating comfort foods doesn't improve mood any faster than eating nothing at all. Cravings may also hit when we are bored or busy and feel the need for stimulation or pleasure. Plus, emotional eating doesn't help you get to the heart of what's eating you.

Food addiction

The types of foods that tend to trigger cravings—the so-called hyperpalatable foods that contain the trifecta of added sugar, salt and fat—often get labeled as "addictive." Although some research suggests that we can develop substance-like addictions to sugar, this is controversial. Sugar has been shown to light up the reward center in the brains, but food is supposed to be rewarding. And that reward response? It's stronger in individuals who are dieting or otherwise restricting sugar. Addiction aside, we're more likely to crave what we can't have. If you categorically deny yourself chocolate, you will probably crave chocolate. If you love a certain food, find a balanced way to include it in your life.

Cravings vs. hunger

It can be challenging to distinguish cravings from true hunger, especially if you aren't in touch with your body's internal hunger cues. Cravings tend to be more specific than hunger, so if you feel like you need to eat, but don't have a particular food in mind, it's probably hunger. If you are laser-focused on one single food, it's probably a craving. Primal hunger plus cravings equal harder-to-resist cravings, which is a pretty good reason to avoid letting yourself get too hungry.

To spot big-picture patterns and hone in on what you're really craving, try keeping a "cravings journal." Instead of cookie every afternoon, you might just really need a break from your desk. That movie popcorn? You could just be operating on autopilot. Instead of ice cream, you might need a hug or a friendly ear to listen to your troubles. Instead of being a slave to your cravings, listen to them and be curious. They may be giving you valuable information—and it might not even be about food.

Finding and feeling hunger

Still not sure how to distinguish between true hunger, cravings or a simple desire to eat? Don't feel bad…it's hard for many people, but with practice you will become more attuned to whether your need to eat is coming from below your neck (true hunger), from your head (craving) or from your mouth (desire to eat, or "mouth hunger"). In her book Bite By Bite, Geneen Roth gives a great example:

You're walking down the street and you pass by a bakery. The instant you do, your brain yells, "I want a cinnamon roll!" Now, you didn't want a cinnamon roll five minutes earlier, but now you urgently want a cinnamon roll. This is clearly not a case of your body telling you what it needs (i.e., it's not true hunger). These signals are coming from above the neck, either from your mouth (because, let's face it, cinnamon rolls are yummy) or from your head (because you developed a sudden craving for sugar or are in need of comfort).

Here are a few examples of how hunger, desire to eat and cravings may feel:

- You haven't eaten for many hours and feel ravenous. Your stomach feels empty and it is probably growing or rumbling. You might feel lightheaded (just make sure you aren't mildly dehydrated). This is hunger.
- You ate a big meal yet you still want to eat dessert. This is a desire to eat.
- You have a very strong urge to eat, accompanied by a feeling of tension and an unpleasant feeling of yearning in your mouth, throat or body. This is a craving.

Using intuitive and mindful eating can help you tell the difference between true hunger…and all the rest.

Before you sit down to eat anything (because you don't stand when you eat, right?), pay attention to how your stomach feels. Rate your hunger on a scale of 0 to 10, with 5 being neutral, 0 being starving and 10 being stuffed. If you are below a 5, it's likely true hunger. Halfway through the meal, notice again how your stomach feels. If you are a 5 or above, you are no longer hungry. Continuing to eat means you are eating because of cravings or because you simply want to eat. If you are still below a 5, you're still truly hungry. Rate your hunger again once you're done eating. Pay attention to your thoughts. Do you want to eat more? Do you feel physical sensations in your stomach, or is it more in your mouth or throat? Do you want to eat specific food (this probably means you are feeling a craving or desire to eat)? Or, will any food do (this may mean you are still hungry). 20 minutes after you're done eating, rate your hunger and assess any body sensations again.

Three tips for cooling down cravings

Your brain is a powerful tool for changing intention (craving) into action (either eating the food or not eating the food). Here are some tips on how to steer your thoughts toward effectively resisting cravings, especially cravings that are more mindless or impulsive:

- **Delay and distract.** Cravings may feel strong, but they tend to weaken quickly. Distract yourself by taking a walk, calling a friend or reading a magazine.
- **Practice not reacting.** This is one part of an exercise from the authors of Intuitive Eating. If you find yourself having a craving, commit to delaying eating the food for 10-15 minutes. Find a comfortable place to sit, close your eyes, and follow your breath as you breathe in and out. If your mind wanders, just bring it back to your breath (you may have to do this repeatedly, and that's OK!).
- **Surf the urge.** Instead of distracting yourself, allow yourself to fully feel your craving, or urge. Imagine the craving like an ocean wave, building, then cresting, then

It's important to note that these activities aren't designed to stop you from eating. What they are designed to do is to help you avoid reacting impulsively to a craving. If, in the end, you decide to eat the food you crave, you'll be in a frame of mind more suited to making a thoughtful, conscious decision.

Food addiction

NO ONE DOUBTS the reality—or seriousness—of addiction to alcohol, tobacco or other drugs, but bring up food addiction and you might get a few eye rolls. However, research suggests that food addiction might be more than just an excuse for overeating.

One conundrum with food addiction is that unlike alcohol or drugs, we need food. We depend on food to live. There's a saying in Overeaters Anonymous: "When you are addicted to alcohol, you put the tiger in the cage and leave it there in order to recover. When you are addicted to food, you put the tiger in the cage but take it out three times a day for a walk."

Who is more likely to experience what feels like food addiction? Adults age 35 or older, women, and people in larger bodies. Perhaps not surprisingly, the foods most often labeled as addictive contain sugar, caffeine or fat. Milkshakes, soda, pizza or French fries are more likely to be addictive —broccoli and salmon are not. When someone goes from wanting soda to needing it, food addiction may be the issue.

Much of the research on food addiction comes out of Yale University, which led to the development of the Yale Food Addiction Scale (YFAS). Brain scans have shown that in people with food addiction, eating addictive foods trigger brain responses that look very similar to responses to alcohol or hard drugs. In one study of women who met the YFAS criteria for food addiction, simply seeing photos of a milkshake caused the areas of the brain associated with craving and motivation to light up. When they actually drank the shake, the area of the brain associated with self-control showed little activity. However, one major limitation of the Yale food addiction research is that they didn't ask the female college-age subjects if they were dieting. Food restriction heightens the brain's reward response to food, especially highly palatable food.

Defining food addiction

The commonly used definition of food addiction takes its cue from drug and alcohol addiction. Someone with a food addiction builds tolerance to the problem food, so that it takes more and more of it to be satisfied, and they experience withdrawal symptoms if they stop eating that food. They are likely to eat larger amounts of the food than intended, and keep doing it even though they know it may be damaging their health. They may devote significant time and energy trying to avoid the food without success. On the other hand, pursuit of that food may take them away from other activities.

Not all overeating is due to food addiction. There are many reasons someone might overeat on a regular basis. Some people tend to eat mindlessly, with little awareness of how much they are eating. Some people eat excessively because of a diagnosable eating disorder, such as binge eating disorder or bulimia nervosa. Some researchers say that food addiction exists, but its more of a behavioral addiction. In other words, it has more in common with, say, gambling addiction than cocaine addiction.

Another perspective

Not all nutrition professionals accept the idea that food is addictive. In fact, there's a concern that labeling someone as a "food addict" (whether that label is self-directed or comes from someone else) makes it a self-fulfilling prophecy: That if you identify as someone who "can't be trusted around cookies" or "can't handle myself around sugar" you will end up acting accordingly. Sometimes our thoughts, and the stories we tell ourselves, become our "reality."

Also, restricting foods (or certain foods), as happens with dieting, can increase the allure of those foods (forbidden fruit syndrome!) as well as obsessive thoughts about those foods, possibly leading to binge-like behavior when resolve cracks, and those foods are consumed.

Finally, it's interesting that while sugar and other hyper palatable foods light up the reward centers (or pleasure centers) of the brain, so do things like holding your child or listening to music you love. Just some food for thought!

Disordered eating

STRESS EATING, EMOTIONAL EATING and comfort eating definitely fall in the broad category of disordered eating. To put that in perspective, typical dieting behaviors like restricting calories to the point of being hungry almost constantly also qualifies as disordered eating. So what's not disordered eating? Refer to the "Normal Eaters" section at the end of Chapter 12.

Someone may have disordered eating patterns, but that doesn't necessarily mean they have an eating disorder. If you have any concerns that you might have or be at risk for an eating disorder, ask yourself these four questions. A yes to two or more could be cause for concern.

- Do you ever eat in secret?
- Do you worry that you have lost control over how much you eat?
- Do you make yourself sick when you feel uncomfortably full?
- Have you ever suffered from an eating disorder?

I've included a link to a free, confidential online screening from the National Eating Disorder Association in the online resource list, but you can also access it right now at www.mybodyscreening.org.

Chapter summary

I often say that when it comes to eating, it's never just about the food. Understanding why you eat is important, especially if you use food for things that food was never meant for (like relieving stress, soothing emotions, staving off boredom).

Here are the main takeaways from Chapter 15:

- People engage in stress and emotional eating because it works—sort of—but it's not a lasting solution.
- Part of coping with cravings involves understanding what it is you're hungry for (it may not be food) and why.
- Emotional eating is a sign that you have deeper needs that deserve tending.
- Food addiction may or may not be a real thing. It also may simply be a label that doesn't really help us.
- Fortunately, most people don't have eating disorders, but many, many people have what could fairly be described as disordered eating.

Next: It's a Wrap

It's a Wrap

WELL, THAT'S IT...FOR NOW. There's always more to say when you're talking about food, nutrition, health, self-care and well-being! Since some of the topics I included in this book are deep topics (really deep), I included a resource list on the next page of books and podcasts I highly recommend. You'll also find this list on HealthyForYourLife.com, and I'll update it as the mood strikes and more worthy books and podcasts come to my attention.

I also write about all of these topics (and more) on my blog and in the freelance articles I do for various publications. You can find all of that at www.nutritionbycarrie.com.

Just a few final reminders:

1. Nutrition doesn't have to be complicated.
2. There are ways to put a nourishing meal on the table that don't require channeling Julia Child (may she rest in peace).
3. If you have a complicated relationship with food, sorting that out is far more important than worrying about how many vegetables you're eating.
4. How we live (food, movement, sleep, stress, social connection) matters far, far more than weight when it comes to health.
5. You are inherently worthy of self-care.

Finally, thanks for reading, and don't forget to visit the book website at www.healthyforyourlife.com for downloads, recommendations for books podcasts, articles and websites to further your journey, and more!

THESE RECIPES AREN'T FANCY OR COMPLICATED, but they are real work-horses in my kitchen. They either provide a base for other recipes, or they pull together always-on-hand staples from my pantry and refrigerator. Their convenience and ease pleases me—and so does their flavor!

Little black dress recipes (aka, the very basics)

How to bake chicken breasts

There are many ways to do this, including some that involve pan searing first, but this is how I do it. You can use boneless chicken breasts or bone-in breasts. Bone-in breasts generally have richer flavor, but boneless is sometimes just easier to deal with, depending on what you plan to do with them.

1. Defrost chicken breasts ahead of time. Don't try to do it in the microwave...trust me. You can take them out a day or two ahead of time and defrost them in the fridge.
2. Move oven rack to middle of oven. Preheat oven to 350 degrees F. This can take about 20 minutes.
3. Pat chicken breasts dry with paper towels. Place in pan or on rimmed baking sheet, "pretty side" up. Rub with olive oil and sprinkle with salt, pepper and seasoning of choice if desired (I often use granulated garlic, a Cajun spice blend or Herbes de Provence).
4. Bake for about 25-30 minutes (boneless) or 35-40 minutes (bone-in). The exact cooking time will depend on the size of the chicken breasts and your oven. Always treat cooking times as guidelines, not hard-and-fast rules. I often set a kitchen timer for 5-15 minutes before I expect something to be done (depending on total estimated cooking time), check it, and put it back in the oven if it needs more time.

So how to you know when your chicken breasts are done? If you have a working meat thermometer, insert it into the center of the thickest part of the breast. It's done when it reaches 160 degrees F. I only ever seem to have working candy thermometers, so instead I take a small, sharp knife and cut into the thick part of the breast. If the juices run clear, and the interior of the flesh doesn't look pink it's done.

Let sit out of the oven for about five minutes before serving or cutting them up.

How to accessorize: I usually bake extra chicken breasts to use for a few days of leftovers. I love them chunked up on a salad or sliced for a sandwich. It's also easy to shred or dice them, mix them with a can of black beans, heat on the stove, then top with salsa, avocado and a little shredded cheese and serve over brown rice and/or shredded cabbage.

How to roast vegetables

Roasting vegetables brings out their natural sweetness and flavor like no other cooking method (grilling comes close).

1. Adjust oven rack to one of the middle positions. Preheat oven to anywhere between 350 and 450 degrees F. A hotter oven is better (and it means a shorter roasting time), but you do have some flexibility in roasting temperatures, which comes in handy if you're also using the oven to cook something that requires a lower temperature.

2. Prepare vegetables. I chunk up thicker veggies like squash, large carrots, cauliflower, whole broccoli heads, potatoes, onions, and peppers, but I leave veggies like asparagus, broccolette (broccoli rabe), slender carrots and green beans whole, just trimming the ends. Try to make the pieces fairly uniform in size, so they are all done at the same time.

3. Put veggies in large bowl and toss with olive oil. Sometimes it's easier to use your hands than a spoon. If you really don't want to get a bowl dirty, you can put the veggies in their pan, drizzle with oil, then use your hands to move the veg around to get them coated.

4. One way or another, put the veggies in a baking dish or a rimmed baking sheet, then sprinkle lightly with salt and pepper.

5. Roast for 10-15 minutes (depending on oven temperature), then remove pan, toss/turn over veggies with a spatula, and return to oven. They'll take another 10-15 minutes, depending. Just keep an eye on them. How done you want them is pretty much personal preference.

How to use: Roasted vegetables are great hot, but they make good leftovers to throw onto a salad, mix with chunks of leftover chicken breast (perhaps tossed with a vinaigrette), or chop further and add to scrambled eggs.

How to make a vinaigrette
(and shun store-bought salad dressing)

I never buy salad dressing anymore. Never. And I eat a LOT of salads. It is soooo easy to make your own, vinaigrette and when you do, you skip out on all the fillers, preservatives, additives and whatnot in the pre-made dressings.

1. Gather a jar with a tight-fitting lid, a tablespoon measure, extra-virgin olive oil, vinegar of choice, salt, pepper, and Dijon mustard if you want to make your vinaigrette French-style.
2. Measure 6 tablespoons olive oil and 2 tablespoons vinegar into the jar. Add a pinch of salt and some fresh ground pepper. Stir in a teaspoon of Dijon mustard if you like. The guideline here is a 3-to-1 ratio of oil to acid (vinegar). You can make as much or as little as you need.
3. Shake the jar vigorously to mix (see why you need a tight-fitting lid?). The dressing will separate as it sits, be-cause it's all real ingredients, no emulsifiers. Just shake it up whenever you're ready to use it.

If I make enough to only last a few days, I usually leave the jar on the counter at room temperature. If it will last longer than that, I store it in the fridge, then take it out to let it "unchill" a bit before I use it. The olive oil won't harden at fridge temp, but it will be less fluid, making it hard to mix it up.

Variations: You can replace some or all of the vinegar with lemon juice. You can add some granulated garlic, or even some minced fresh garlic if you have the time and inclination.

Pantry staple recipes

Tuna and white bean salad
Serves 2

This is one of my all-time favorite pantry staple recipes. It has saved my bacon more than once when I had no idea what to make for a work lunch.

- Drain and rinse one can of white beans. Put in bowl.
- Drain one can of tuna. Use a fork to flake it into the bowl.
- Toss in a few tablespoons of capers or quartered Kalamata olives.
- Add vinaigrette (or olive oil and vinegar) and salt and pepper to taste.
- Serve on bed of lettuce.

How easy is that? Very easy. You can easily ramp it up a bit by adding some walnut halves, cherry tomatoes, diced roasted red peppers. You can use lemon juice instead of vinegar. It's delicious!

Wheatberry, chickpea and chicken salad
Serves 3-4

Grains and beans make a great base for salads (they pack really well for lunches). Here's a concoction I sometimes throw together for lunches:

- Put cooked wheatberries in bowl.*
- Drain one can of chickpeas, add to bowl.
- Dice leftover grilled or baked chicken breasts or thighs, put in bowl.
- Quarter some Kalamata olives, add to bowl.
- Sprinkle in some feta cheese (you don't need much, because it's so flavorful).
- Add vinaigrette or oil and vinegar, and toss to combine.

* Put ¾ cup wheatberries with 3 cups water (1:4 ratio) into a small pot, covered. Bring to a boil then reduce to a simmer. They will probably take about 40 minutes, but check for doneness at 30 minutes by bite testing. (When fully cooked, wheatberries will be chewy and firm, but not hard to chew.) Drain when done.

Stovetop oatmeal
Serves 1

I dislike instant oatmeal packets with a passion. They are gummy, overly sweet...and it's easy and quick to make my own:

- Add ⅓ cup oatmeal (regular or thick) and ⅔ cups liquid (1:2 ratio) per person to a pot (smaller pot for fewer portions) over medium heat.
- Add a pinch of salt. I also like to add vanilla extract and cinnamon, and sometimes a pinch of nutmeg.
- Stir to combine as you add things, but you can mostly leave it alone until it starts to bubble. When it does, turn down the heat to a simmer, and start stirring. Sometimes I stir a little, sometimes a lot. I'm not sure that it matters! Just make sure it's simmering instead of boiling and spewing.
- Cook until it has the consistency you like, and serve.

I rarely use sweeteners in my oatmeal, so I often add some chopped ripe banana or some dried raisins or other dried fruit. I may also add some unsweetened shredded coconut and a few nuts or a small dollop of nut butter (peanut or almond). Sometimes I do sweeten it slightly—a touch of Trader Joe's pumpkin butter or a drizzle of maple syrup are my favorites.

Mediterranean recipes

Farro & arugula salad with pistachios
Serves 4-6

1 cup farro
2 teaspoons kosher salt
2 small bay leaves, or one large
6 tablespoons extra-virgin olive oil
2 tablespoons fresh lemon juice
½ cup crumbled feta cheese
½ cup shelled pistachio nuts (or substitute chopped wal-
    nuts or almonds)
½ cup chopped dried apricots
3 cups baby arugula leaves (or three big handfuls)
2 cups coarsely chopped herbs: parsley, cilantro and mint
Sea salt to taste

1. In a medium saucepan, bring farro, salt, bay leaves and three
   cups water to a simmer. Continue to simmer uncovered until
   farro is tender and liquid evaporates, about 30 minutes. If
   liquid evaporates before the farro is done, add a bit more. If
   the farro is done but there is liquid remaining, pour off the
   excess. Let the farro cool, then remove the bay leaves.
2. In a medium or large salad bowl, combine the olive oil, lemon juice and a pinch of sea salt. Whisk to mix.
3. Add the farro, pistachios and feta cheese and stir to mix well.
4. Just before serving, fold in the chopped herbs, arugula and
   additional salt (if needed).

Mediterranean chickpea salad

Serves 2-4

This simple salad includes many foods that are central to the Mediterranean diet and is lovely on its own or as a side dish.

1 15-ounce can chickpeas, rinsed and drained, or 2 cups
    cooked chickpeas (from dried)
⅓ cup chopped or quartered Kalamata olives
¼ cup chopped almonds
2 ounces feta cheese, crumbled
½ cup chopped fresh flat-leaf (Italian) parsley
    2 tablespoons fresh lemon juice
    2 tablespoons extra-virgin olive oil
    1 small garlic clove, minced or pressed
    Sea salt and freshly ground pepper to taste

1. Place chickpeas, olives, almonds, feta and parsley in a medium bowl. Toss gently to combine.
2. Add lemon juice, olive oil and garlic to bowl, toss again to coat. Taste and add salt and pepper as needed.
3. Serve immediately or cover and refrigerate. Can be served chilled or at room temperature.

ACKNOWLEDGEMENTS

THANK YOU TO MY patients, clients and readers, who inspire me to learn more and do better every single day. Thank you to my many, many mentors (some of whom have no idea I consider them mentors), who help me learn more and do better every single day! Thank you to my editors at the various publications I write for, who give me an outlet for doing deep dives into nutrition research then shaping what I learn into something helpful for my peers and/or everyday people who like reading about nutrition. Thank you to my husband, Jeff, for always being there for me, even when I'm overextended and a little (ahem) stressed. And I want to thank myself for not giving up on the idea of going back to graduate school to study nutrition, even though that little voice inside my head told me, "Two years of science classes before you even apply to grad school? You can't do that...you're a writer, not a 'science person.'" Turns out that little voice was wrong...science is fun, and my journalism career is a million times more fulfilling now that I get to write about nutrition, food and food relationships all the time.

Made in the USA
Monee, IL
13 December 2019